Good Housekeeping Express

Good Housekeeping would like to dedicate this book to the late Steve Baxter, a hugely talented photographer who we had the pleasure of working with over the years and who photographed many of the beautiful images within *Good Housekeeping Express* and for *Good Housekeeping* magazine. He was a true joy to work with and is sadly missed.

HarperCollins*Publishers*
1 London Bridge Street
London SE1 9GF

www.harpercollins.co.uk

First published by HarperCollins*Publishers* 2019

10 9 8 7 6 5 4 3 2 1

Text and photography © Good Housekeeping 2019
Cover photography © Mike English
Cover food styling: Meike Beck
Cover prop styling: Olivia Wardle

Project editors: Lucy Jessop and Georgina Atsiaris

Recipe writers: Meike Beck, Lucy Jessop, Elizabeth Fox, Sophie Austen-Smith, Monaz Dumasia, Charlotte Watson, Suzannah Butcher, Madeline Burkitt, Olivia Spurrell, Alice Shields, Emma Franklin, Gabriella English

Photographers: Steve Baxter, Kris Kirkham, Maja Smend, Vinny Whiteman, Alex Luck, Martin Poole, Myles New, Sam Stowell, Gareth Morgans, Charlie Richards, Jon Whitaker, Stuart West, Kate Whitaker, Emma Lee, Adrian Lawrence, Mike English, Lara Holmes, Anita Bean

HB ISBN 978-0-00-835789-4

EB ISBN 978-0-00-835790-0

Printed and bound by GPS Group

MIX
Paper from
responsible sources
FSC www.fsc.org **FSC™ C007454**

This book is produced from independently certified FSC™ paper to ensure responsible forest management.

For more information visit: www.harpercollins.co.uk/green

Good Housekeeping

Express

130 delicious recipes in 30 minutes

HarperCollins*Publishers*

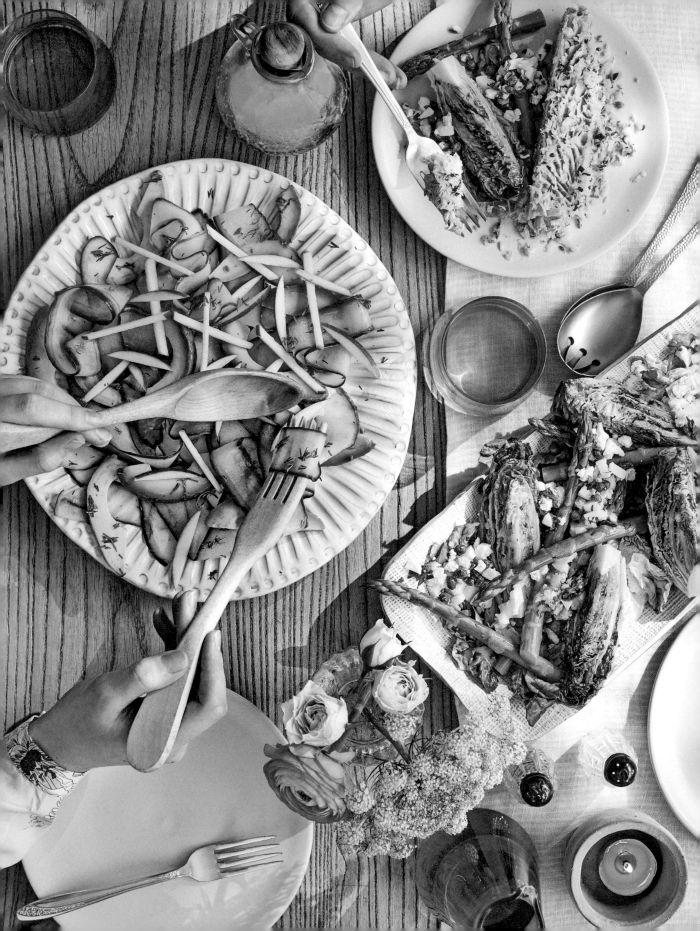

Contents

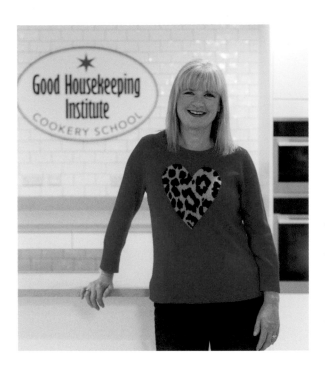

Foreword by Gaby Huddart, Editor-in-Chief

I think we can all agree, it's both the privilege and the curse of our times that we're all more time poor than we'd like to be. New technology, internationalisation and changes in society may have brought us a myriad of benefits but they have also, undoubtedly, added to the epidemic of busyness! It's common to feel that we don't have enough hours in the day or days in the week to achieve all we want to. Who doesn't sometimes get that sense of running just to stand still? So never before has it been more important to cook in a hurry – and not just food to fill us up, but really good, flavoursome, nutritious meals that fuel our frenetic lifestyles and give us pleasure.

At *Good Housekeeping*, though we certainly come up with showstopper menus for those occasions when you're entertaining family and friends and have time to dedicate to the task, we're equally as committed to creating absolutely brilliant recipes for days when you have just 30 minutes (or less) to spare to put a delicious dinner on the table. We make it our mission to come up with meals that you can create from start to finish in pretty much the same time you would wait for a ready meal to cook in the oven! And you'll find the results far tastier and more satisfying.

How do we do it? I wish I could say the process of recipe development is as speedy as the recipes in this book! But, in fact, it's a very rigorous and lengthy process that involves quite a number of us at *Good Housekeeping*.

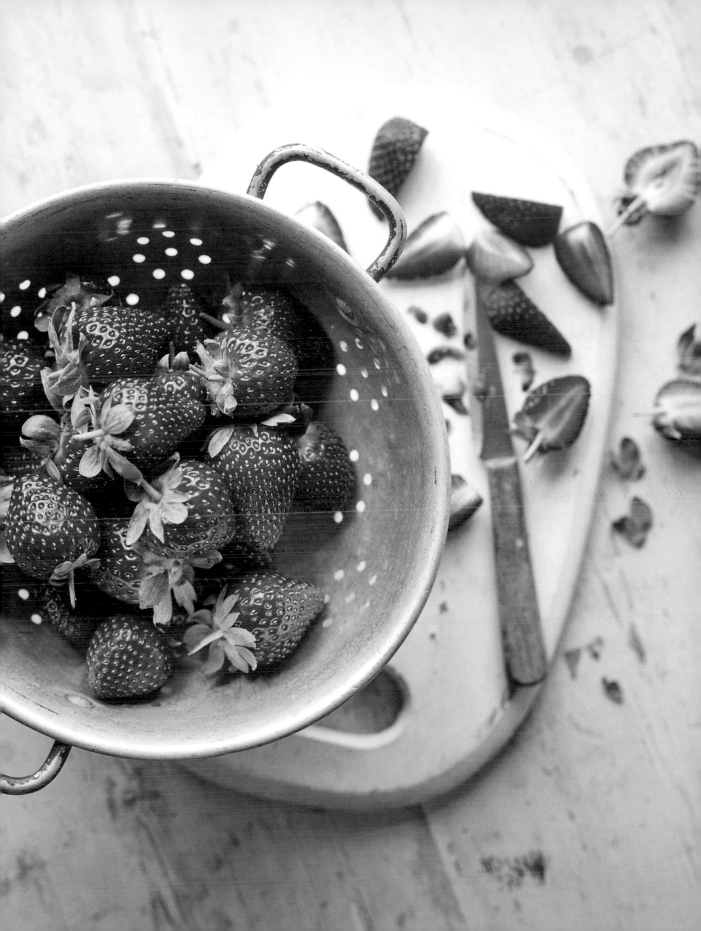

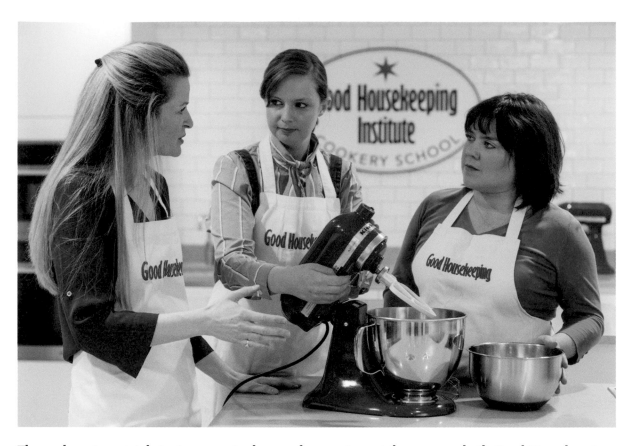

The cookery team triple tests every single one of our recipes at the purpose-built Good Housekeeping Institute in London (from left: Cookery Director Meike Beck, Cookery Writer Alice Shields and Cookery Editor Emma Franklin)

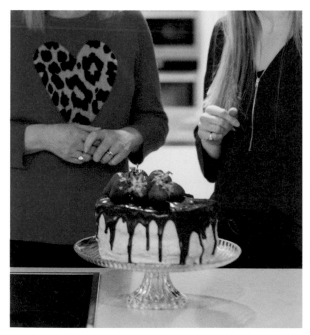

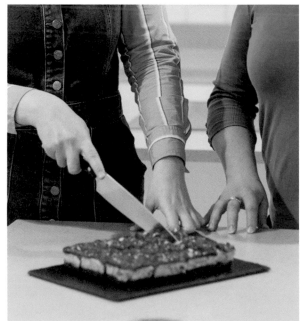

It all starts when cookery director Meike Beck and I get together for a planning meeting and agree on a particular theme for a cookery feature and photoshoot. This will be influenced by factors such as seasonality and availability of ingredients, plus lifestyle trends that we're seeing. For instance, with cuisines such as Thai, Vietnamese and Mexican all noticeably growing in popularity, we know we need to come up with recipes for *Good Housekeeping* readers to reflect these. We also know that we need to balance the number of dishes based on meat and fish and vegetables; with a growing number of readers now vegetarian and vegan and wanting inspiration, we always ensure we come up with great ideas for them. Front of mind, too, is the growth of food intolerances and dietary requirements, so we are constantly aiming to meet the needs of those who need to eat gluten or dairy-free. And we also know that not every household contains precisely the same number of folk, so with a growing number of people living solo, we make sure to create fabulous meals for them, along with larger families.

With the initial concept for a shoot agreed, Meike will brief her cookery team, who all then individually come up with ideas for recipes to fit the theme. Every member of her team is professionally trained and their culinary knowledge is, quite simply, top class. They'll then meet together and thrash out which recipes should make the cut and go into

development, dividing between them for the next stage, where they thoroughly research each dish and write the first draft.

On some magical occasions, the dish can be perfect the very first time it's cooked; but, more often, it will take several tests to get it to the level they're happy with for it to pass the 'first' test stage. This includes the team testing a dish for instructions on how to get ahead, freeze ahead and store it, too. So, if we say that a cake can be stored for five days, for instance, it is checked and eaten on every day for each of the five days. Similarly, if we give a tip on a spice blend, the team has made that blend and checked it, how much to use and how long it will store for.

Absolutely nothing is left to chance by the team, so once a recipe is felt to be sound, it is then passed to a different member of the team to be second tested with all the others that fall into the same photoshoot. At this stage, along with several other members of the *Good Housekeeping* team, I'm fortunate enough to taste the dishes and we discuss whether there are any improvements that could or should be made (happily a very rare occurrence!).

On the day of the shoot itself, the dish undergoes yet another full test and the recipe is followed to the letter by the person cooking it. I promise you, there's absolutely no trickery in any of the photos in this book. If you see how it looks, that's the result you should be able to get, too.

One point that's worth making in terms of the timing on our recipes is that we feel

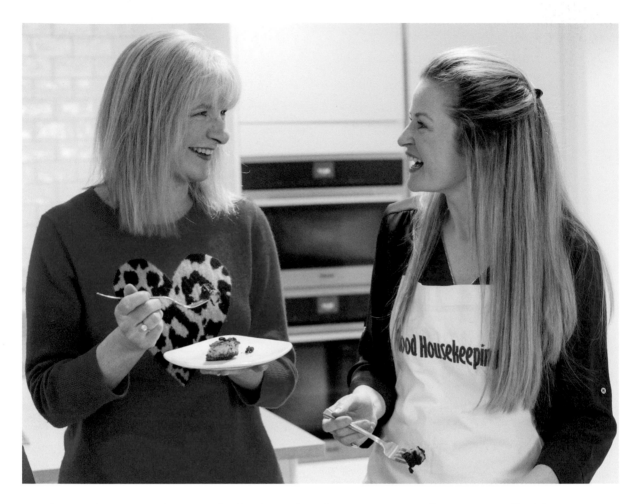

Good Housekeeping's Editor-in-Chief Gaby and Cookery Director Meike taste test all of the recipes – it's one of the perks of the job!

you can multi-task. So, while, for instance, you may be frying an onion, we think it's possible for you to be chopping some herbs or other vegetables. If you do this, all the recipes in this book can be completed in 30 minutes or less – we know because we've triple tested them!

I do hope you find inspiration in this book and find it an invaluable helping hand in your kitchen. I know that since I've worked at *Good Housekeeping*, my own repertoire of midweek meals has improved

exponentially thanks to the fantastic recipes conjured by Meike and the cookery team – and this is a superb collection of them. I know my own family will be forever thankful for the injection of *Good Housekeeping* culinary know-how into our lives and I sincerely hope that yours will be, too.

Enjoy!

Gaby

The Measurements

°C	Fan Oven	Gas mark
110	90	¼
130	110	½
140	120	1
150	130	2
170	150	3
180	160	4
190	170	5
200	180	6
220	200	7
230	210	8
240	220	9

WEIGHTS

Metric	Imperial
15g	½oz
25g	1oz
40g	1½oz
50g	2oz
75g	3oz
100g	3½oz
125g	4oz
150g	5oz
175g	6oz
200g	7oz
225g	8oz
250g	9oz
275g	10oz
300g	11oz
350g	12oz
375g	13oz
400g	14oz
425g	15oz
450g	1lb
550g	1¼lb
700g	1½lb
900g	2lb
1.1kg	2½lb

VOLUMES

Metric	Imperial
5ml	1 tsp
15ml	1 tbsp
25ml	1fl oz
50ml	2fl oz
100ml	3½fl oz
125ml	4fl oz
150ml	5fl oz (¼ pint)
175ml	6fl oz
200ml	7fl oz
250ml	9fl oz
300ml	10fl oz (½ pint)
500ml	17fl oz
600ml	1 pint
900ml	1½ pints
1 litre	1¾ pints
2 litres	3½ pints

LENGTHS

Metric	Imperial
5mm	¼in
1cm	½in
2cm	¾in
2.5cm	1in
3cm	1¼in
4cm	1½in
5cm	2in
7.5cm	3in
10cm	4in
15cm	6in
18cm	7in
20.5cm	8in
23cm	9in
25.5cm	10in
28cm	11in
30.5cm	12in

ALWAYS REMEMBER

- Use one set of measurements – never mix metric and imperial.
- Ovens and grills must be preheated to the specified temperature before cooking.
- All spoon measures are for calibrated measuring spoons, and should be level, unless otherwise stated.
- Eggs are medium and free-range and butter is salted, unless otherwise stated.
- Always buy the best-quality meat you can afford.

Dietary Index

Dairy-free recipes

Gluten-free recipes

Vegetarian recipes

Vegan recipes

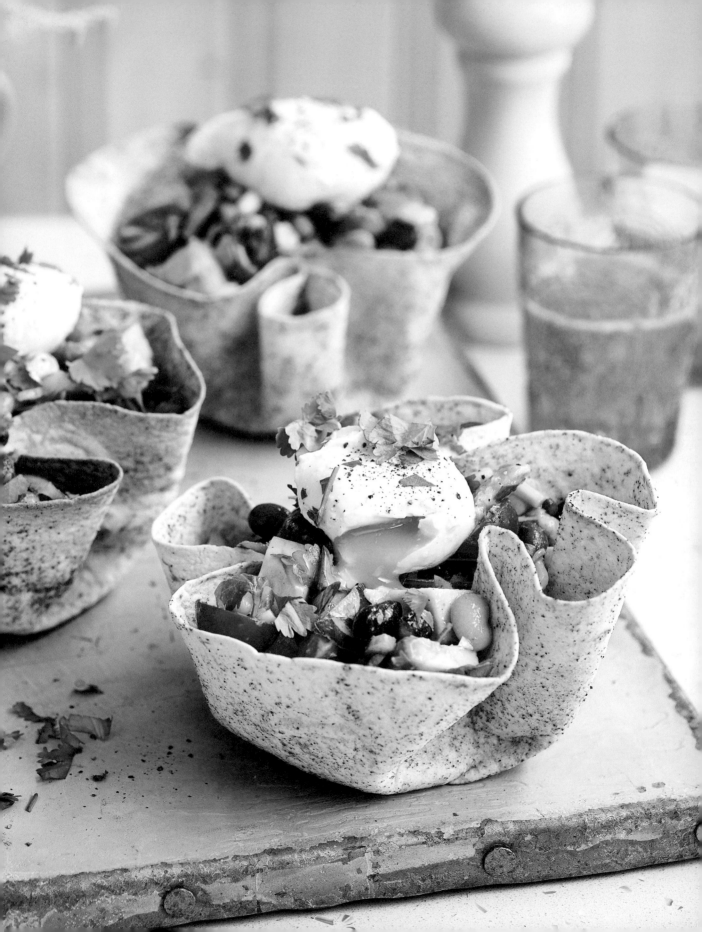

Breakfast and Brunch

Açai Berry Blast Smoothie Bowl

Açai berries are rich in antioxidants. Keep some açai powder in the storecupboard, and you can give any smoothie an instant boost.

Hands-on time: 5 minutes
Serves 1

50ml (2fl oz) milk
1 frozen chopped banana
1 tbsp açai powder
75g (3oz) strawberries
75g (3oz) blueberries
1 tsp honey
Extra fruit, chopped pistachio
   kernals and coconut flakes,
   to serve (optional)

PER SERVING 318cals,
2g protein, 3g fat (2g
saturates), 14g carbs (12g
total sugars), 3g fibre

1. In a blender, whiz together the milk, chopped banana, açai powder, strawberries, blueberries and the honey. Transfer to a bowl and top with extra fruit, chopped pistachios and coconut flakes, if you like.

Green Goddess Smoothie Bowl

Give your potassium levels a boost with this zingy smoothie.

Hands-on time: 5 minutes
Serves 1

75ml (3fl oz) apple juice
1 frozen chopped banana, plus
   extra to serve (optional)
Juice of ½ lime
Large handful of spinach
¼ avocado
100g (3½oz) pineapple, plus
   extra to serve (optional)
Vegan granola, to serve
   (optional)

PER SERVING 281cals,
3g protein, 9g fat (2g
saturates), 45g carbs (41g
total sugars), 6g fibre

1. In a blender, whiz together the apple juice, chopped banana, lime juice, spinach, avocado and pineapple. Transfer to a bowl and top with extra pineapple, banana and granola, if you like.

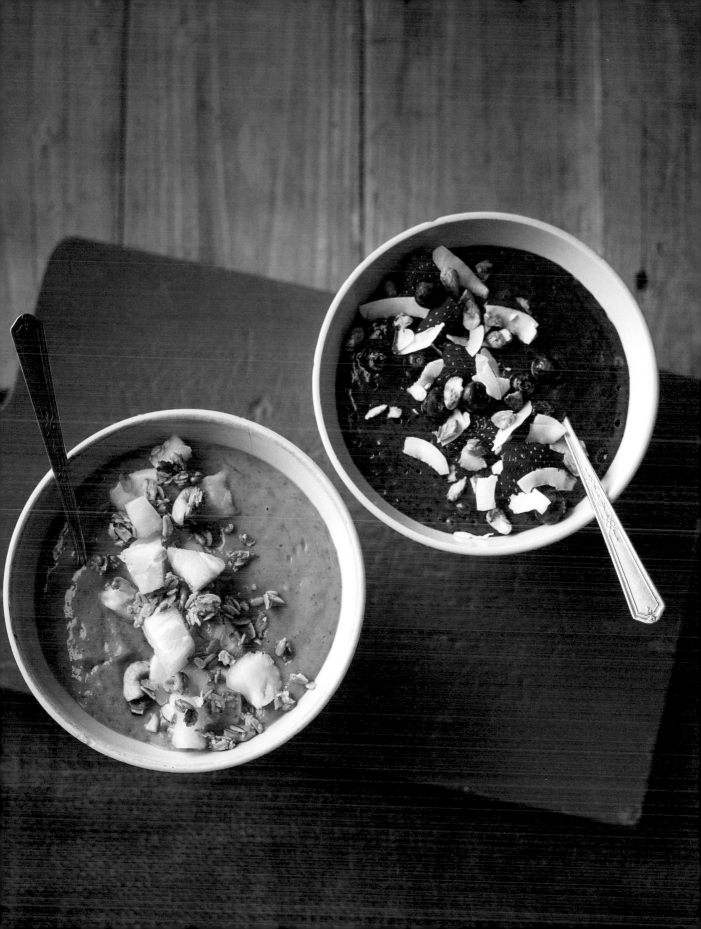

Crunchy Granola and Yogurt Pots

It's easy to adapt this versatile granola to include your favourite dried fruits, nuts or seeds.

Hands-on time: 10 minutes
Cooking time: about
  22 minutes
Serves 18–20 (makes about
  750g/1lb 11oz)

300g (11oz) jumbo
  porridge oats
100g (3½oz) oat or wheat bran
50g (2oz) flaked almonds
25g (1oz) each sesame and
  sunflower seeds
4 tbsp sunflower oil
3 tbsp runny honey
75g (3oz) light brown
  soft sugar
1 tsp vanilla extract
150g (5oz) raisins

TO SERVE (FOR EACH POT)
40g (1½oz) granola
125g (4oz) 0% fat Greek yogurt
50g (2oz) berries
2 tsp runny honey

PER SERVING (as a pot with
yogurt, berries and honey)
266cals, 11g protein, 6g fat
(1g saturates), 43g carbs
(31g total sugars), 4g fibre

1. Preheat the oven to 200°C (180°C fan) mark 6. In a large bowl, stir together the porridge oats, oat or wheat bran, almonds and seeds.

2. In a small pan set over a medium heat, bring the oil, honey and sugar to the boil, stirring often until combined. Remove from the heat, stir in the vanilla, then pour the mixture into the dry ingredients and stir to combine.

3. Divide the oat mixture between two baking trays and spread into an even layer. Bake for 15–20 minutes, stirring halfway through, until golden. Remove the granola from the oven and spread it out on to a couple of large plates. Cool. Sprinkle over the raisins, then transfer the granola to an airtight container.

4. Serve the granola in pots layered with yogurt, berries and honey.

● GH TIP
Store the cooled granola in an airtight container for up to a month.

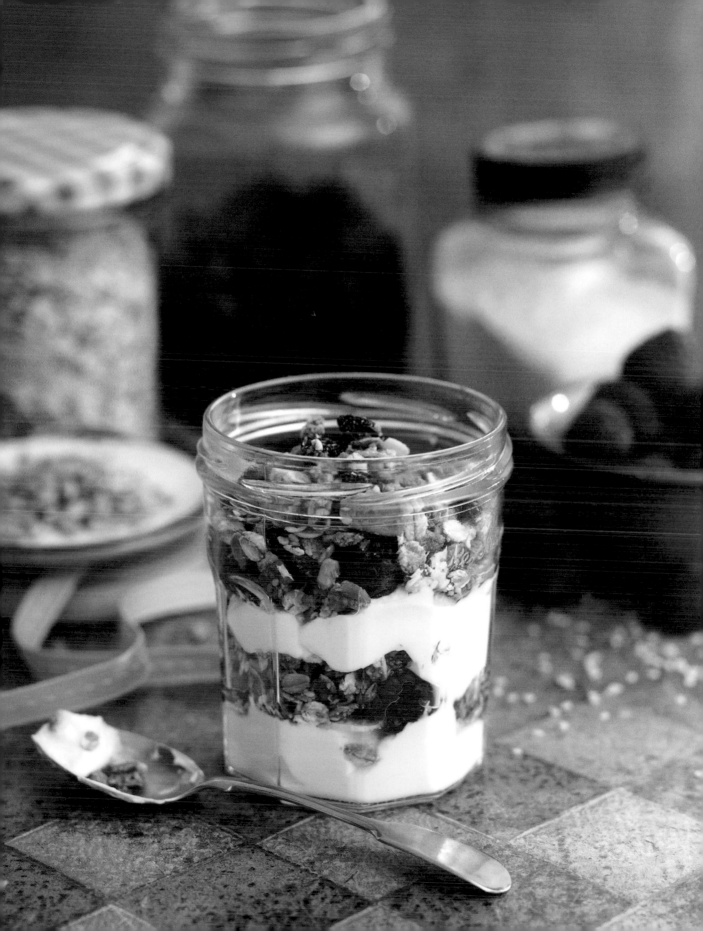

BREAKFAST BEVERAGES

Cooking up a celebratory brunch or after a healthy start to the day? Choose from the classic, spiced Bloody Mary, an indulgent Kahlua-laced cocktail for coffee lovers or a healthy, vitamin-packed berry smoothie to drink alongside your weekend brunch.

The Best Bloody Mary

Hands-on time: 5 minutes
Serves 6 (makes about 1 litre/1¾ pints)

PER SERVING 74cals, 1g protein, 0g fat (0g saturates), 4g carbs (4g total sugars), 1g fibre

150ml (5fl oz) vodka
800ml (1⅓ pints) tomato juice
½ tsp Worcestershire sauce, plus extra to serve
¼–½ tsp Tabasco sauce (to taste), plus extra to serve
½ tsp celery salt
6 sticks celery

1. Pour the vodka and tomato juice into a large jug. Stir in the Worcestershire sauce, Tabasco sauce (to taste), celery salt and a little freshly ground pepper.

2. To serve, fill 6 tall glasses with ice cubes and add a celery stick to each. Divide the tomato mixture among the glasses. Serve with Tabasco, Worcestershire sauce and celery salt alongside for guests to customise their drinks.

Coffee Kicker

Hands-on time: 5 minutes
Serves 8 (makes about 900ml/1½ pints)

PER SERVING (with 1 tsp cream) 69cals, 0g protein, 3g fat (2g saturates), 10g carbs (10g total sugars), 0g fibre

700ml (1¼ pints) strong filter coffee
3 tbsp Kahlua or other coffee liqueur
4 tbsp caster sugar (to taste)
Lightly whipped double cream, to serve
Cocoa powder, to dust

1. Pour the coffee into a jug with Kahlua or other coffee liqueur and caster sugar to taste. Mix well. Pour into small glass coffee cups and top with a dollop of whipped double cream and a light dusting of cocoa powder.

Strawberry and Banana Smoothie

Hands-on time: 5 minutes
Serves 4 (makes 800ml/1⅓ pints)

PER SERVING 112cals, 4g protein, 1g fat (1g saturates), 22g carbs (21g total sugars), 1g fibre

2 ripe bananas, roughly chopped
12 hulled strawberries
200ml (7fl oz) semi-skimmed milk
100g (3½oz) vanilla or strawberry yogurt
Honey, to taste

1. Put the bananas, strawberries, milk and yogurt in a blender. Blend until smooth, adding a bit more milk if the mixture seems too thick. Add honey to taste, then divide among 4 glasses and serve.

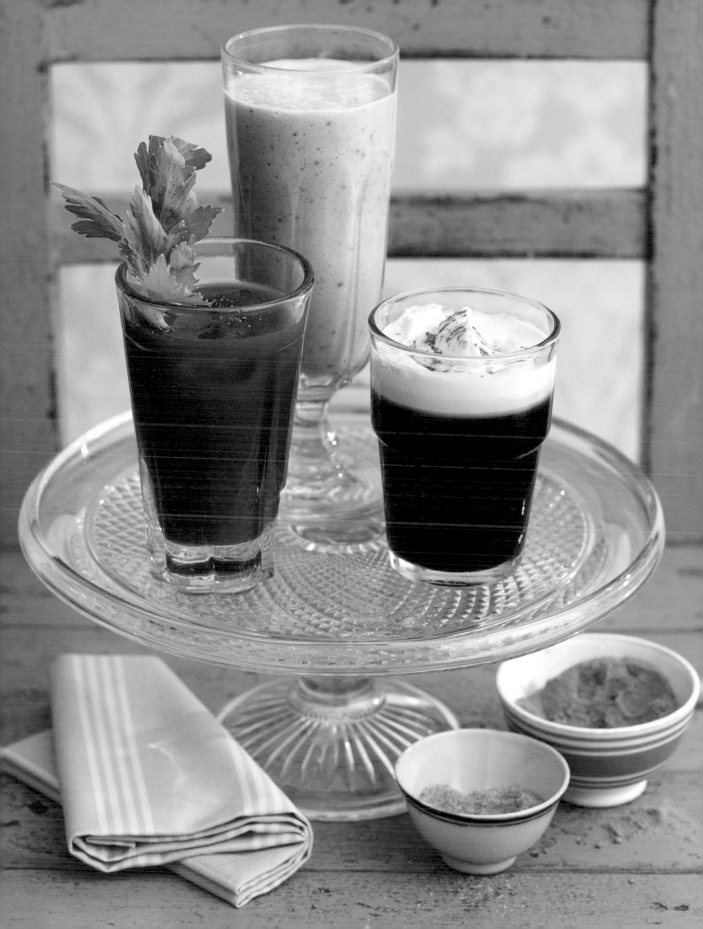

Coconut and Pomegranate Chia Seed Pudding

Chia seeds are a brilliant source of vegetarian protein, and will thicken milk to a yogurt-like consistency.

Hands-on time: 5 minutes, plus chilling
Serves 4

400ml (14fl oz) coconut milk
2 tbsp maple syrup
8 tbsp chia seeds
50ml (2fl oz) milk
Small handful of pomegranate seeds, to serve

PER SERVING 361cals, 9g protein, 28g fat (15g saturates), 15g carbs (7g total sugars), 9g fibre

1. In a large bowl, mix together the coconut milk, maple syrup and chia seeds. Chill for 15 minutes.

2. Take out of the fridge and stir through the milk. Divide the pudding among 4 x 150ml (5fl oz) glasses. Top each with a few pomegranate seeds and serve.

● GH TIP
To make this dairy free and vegan, swap the cow's milk for oat, soya or almond milk.

Super Chias

These little black or white seeds are packed with protein, fibre, omega-3 oils, iron, calcium, magnesium and antioxidants. If you haven't tried them, you could be missing a real health trick. Gram for gram they are higher in omega-3 than salmon and just 2 tablespoons of the seeds provide a third of your daily fibre needs. Add them to smoothies, salads, porridge, granola or baked goods.

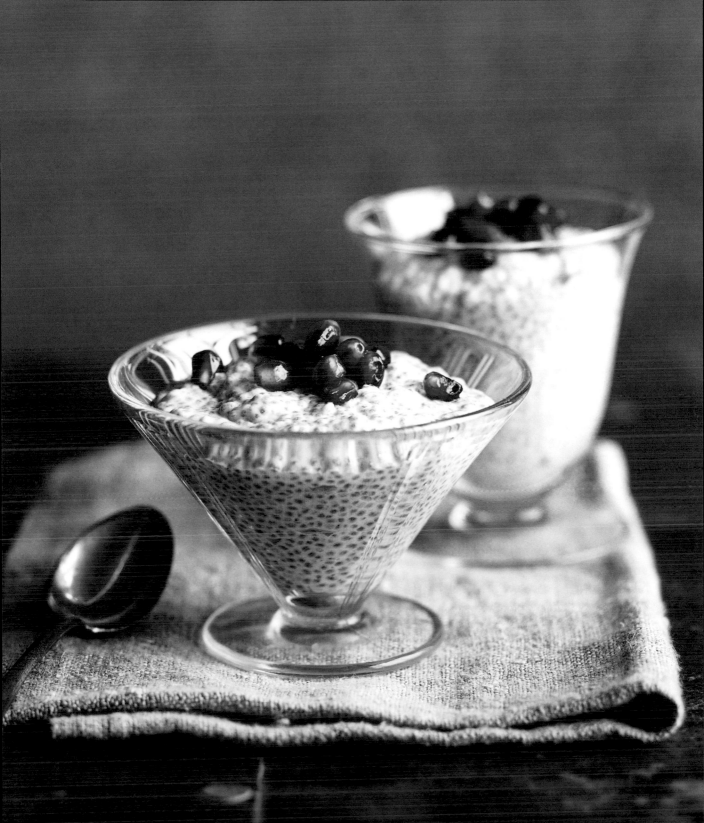

Spiced Rhubarb French Toast

Tender pink shoots of forced rhubarb are in season in the UK from February to early May. They're delicious with this French toast for a weekend brunch or with yogurt and granola for a fast and healthy weekday alternative.

Hands-on time: 20 minutes
Cooking time: 15 minutes
Serves 6

2 medium eggs
150ml (¼ pint) milk
1 tsp vanilla extract
1 tbsp caster sugar
Knob of butter, to fry
6 thick slices of brioche (taken from a loaf)
Icing sugar, to dust
4 tbsp crème fraîche
Zest of 1 orange, to serve

FOR THE RHUBARB COMPOTE
50g (2oz) caster sugar
10 crushed cardamom pods
Finely grated zest and juice of 2 oranges
400g (14oz) forced rhubarb, cut into 5cm (2in) lengths

PER SERVING 287cals, 7g protein, 12g fat (7g saturates), 35g carbs (21g total sugars), 2g fibre

1. For the compote, gently heat the sugar, cardamom pods and the orange zest and juice in a large frying pan with 2 tablespoons water until the sugar has dissolved. Simmer for 2–3 minutes. Strain the syrup, discarding the pods, then return to the pan and add the rhubarb, spreading it out in a single layer. Cook the rhubarb pieces over a low heat for 3–5 minutes, turning them halfway, until completely tender but still holding their shape. Tip out of the pan on to a plate to cool.

2. Meanwhile, whisk together the eggs, milk, vanilla and sugar in a wide shallow bowl. Put the butter in a large, non-stick frying pan set over low to medium heat. Working one slice at a time, dip the brioche into the egg mixture to soak, then add it to the frying pan (do this in batches if your pan isn't big enough). Fry the slices until golden on both sides. Repeat with the remaining brioche.

3. Slice a fried brioche in half, dust with icing sugar and serve with the rhubarb, a dollop of crème fraîche and a little orange zest.

◆ GET AHEAD
Make the rhubarb compote up to a day ahead, then cool, cover and chill.

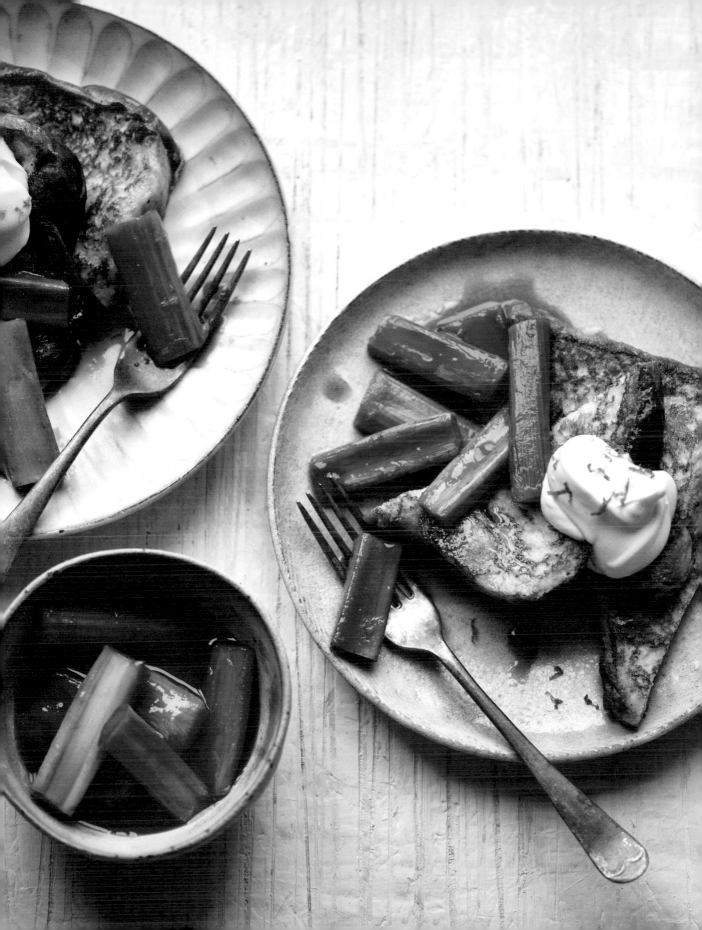

Brandy Mushrooms on Toast

Mushrooms pair so well with thyme, and adding a splash of double cream and brandy makes this dish a real treat. It will taste even better during the autumn, when homegrown mushrooms are in season. Serve with a poached or fried egg on top, if you like.

Hands-on time: 10 minutes
Cooking time: about
   15 minutes
Serves 8

1½ tbsp olive oil
3 shallots, finely sliced
1 garlic clove, sliced
50g (2oz) butter
700g (1½lb) mixed
   mushrooms, such as
   crimini, chestnut and
   portobello
2 tbsp brandy
3 tbsp double cream
½ tbsp fresh lemon
   thyme leaves
1 tbsp chopped fresh parsley,
   plus extra to garnish
8 slices ciabatta

PER SERVING 199cals,
5g protein, 11g fat (6g
saturates), 13g carbs (1g
total sugars), 2g fibre

1. Heat 1 tablespoon of oil in a large frying pan and cook the shallots and garlic gently for 5 minutes until softened. Add 25g (1oz) of the butter and, when it starts to foam, tip in half the mushrooms. Fry over a high heat until browned and the liquid has evaporated. Remove from the pan and set aside. Cook the rest of the mushrooms in the remaining butter.

2. Return the first mushroom and shallot mixture to the pan and pour the brandy on top. Carefully light the liquid with a match to burn off the alcohol, then let the flames die down. Stir in the cream, thyme leaves and parsley, then heat for 2 minutes until bubbling.

3. Meanwhile, heat a griddle pan until hot. Brush the ciabatta slices with the remaining oil and toast them on both sides. Divide the ciabatta among 8 plates, top with the mushroom mixture and garnish with the extra parsley. Serve immediately.

● GH TIP
Make it luxe – add a drizzle of truffle oil to the mushrooms at the end of cooking.

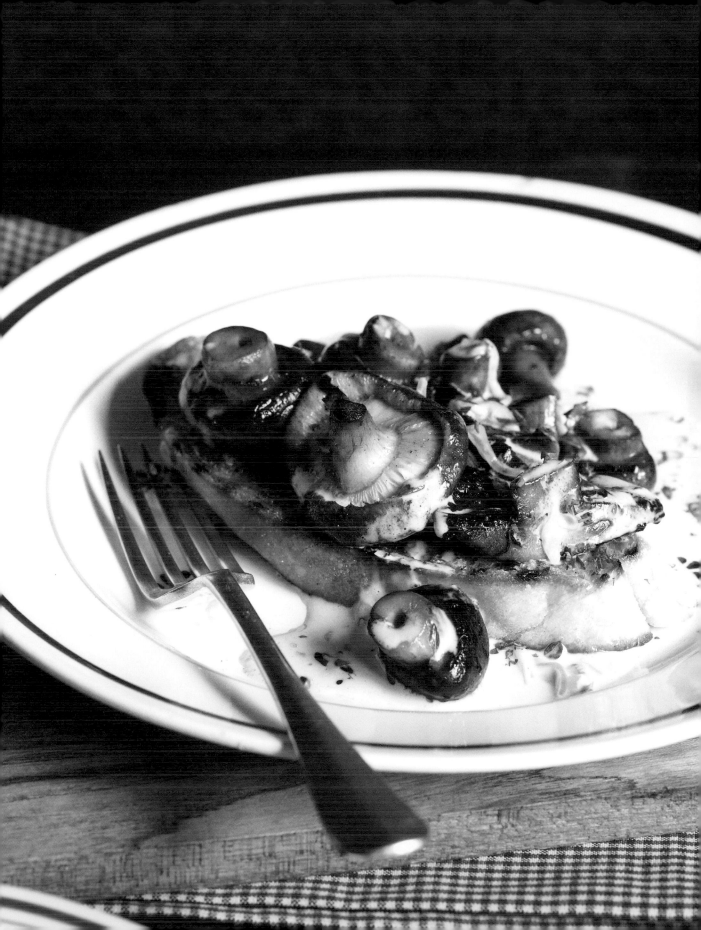

Stuffed Chocolate Pain Perdu with Salted Caramel

Pain perdu (or 'lost bread') is a great way to use up bread that is going stale. We've used brioche for added indulgence, but this tempting recipe also works well with thick-sliced white bread.

Hands-on time: 15 minutes
Cooking time: about
10 minutes
Serves 2

1 medium egg
100ml (3½fl oz) milk
15g (½oz) caster sugar
2 tbsp chocolate hazelnut
    spread
4 slices brioche bread
25g (1oz) unsalted butter
Icing sugar, to dust
Vanilla ice cream, to serve
    (optional)

FOR THE SALTED
CARAMEL
15g (½oz) unsalted butter
25g (1oz) light brown
    soft sugar
75ml (3fl oz) double cream

**PER SERVING (without ice
cream) 750cals, 11g protein,
51g fat (29g saturates), 60g
carbs (37g total sugars), 1g
fibre**

1. To make the salted caramel, heat the butter, sugar and cream in a small pan until melted and smooth. Leave to bubble, stirring frequently, until it reaches a nice golden colour. Take off the heat and add a little salt to taste. Set aside in the pan.

2. In a shallow bowl, whisk together the egg, milk and caster sugar. Spread chocolate hazelnut spread over 2 of the brioche slices, then top each with one of the remaining slices.

3. Dip the brioche sandwiches in the egg mixture on both sides.

4. Put the butter in a large frying pan set over low-medium heat. Fry the soaked sandwiches for a couple of minutes until golden on the base. Flip and fry again until golden on the other side.

5. Meanwhile, gently reheat the salted caramel, then transfer it to a serving bowl. Dust the pain perdu with icing sugar and serve with the salted caramel to drizzle over, plus vanilla ice cream, if you like.

◆ GET AHEAD
Prepare the salted caramel to the end of step 1 up to 2 hours ahead. Complete the recipe to serve.

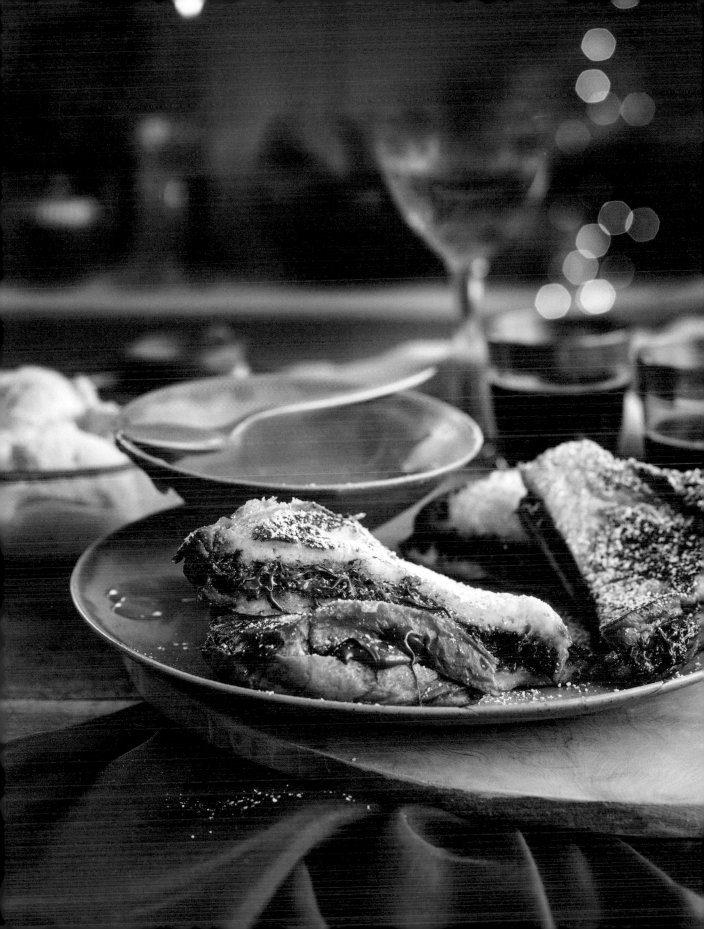

Fluffy American-style Pancakes with Bacon and Maple Syrup

This recipe makes 12 pancakes, so will stretch to serve 6 if you're serving smaller portions or adding lots of extras.

Hands-on time: 20 minutes
Cooking time: about
20 minutes
Serves 4 (makes
12 pancakes)

300g (11oz) self-raising flour
1 tsp baking powder
25g (1oz) caster sugar
2 large eggs
75g (3oz) natural yogurt
300ml (½ pint) semi-skimmed
   milk
40g (1½oz) butter
12 rashers unsmoked
   streaky bacon
75g (3oz) golden syrup
25g (1oz) maple syrup

PER SERVING (for 4)
698cals, 25g protein, 30g fat
(13g saturates), 87g carbs
(31g total sugars), 2g fibre

1. Preheat the oven to 110°C (90°C fan) mark ¼ to use for warming. Sift the flour, baking powder and sugar into a large bowl and stir to combine. In a large jug, whisk the eggs, yogurt and milk together until smooth. Using the whisk, gently stir the wet ingredients into the dry ones until just combined. (The mixture may be a little lumpy, but don't worry!)

2. Heat a knob of the butter in a large frying pan until foaming, then drop large spoonfuls of batter into the pan, spacing them apart (cook in batches). Cook the pancakes for 2–3 minutes until the underside is golden and the tops look dry and bubbly, then flip and cook for a further 2–3 minutes until golden. Put the cooked pancakes on a baking tray, cover with foil and keep warm in the oven. Repeat with the remaining batter.

3. Meanwhile, fry the bacon in a large, non-stick frying pan until crisp and golden.

4. In a small jug or serving bowl, stir together the maple and golden syrups. Serve the warm pancakes stacked with the bacon and drizzled with syrup.

● GH TIP
Mixing golden syrup with maple syrup will save you money, as pure maple syrup is quite expensive. If you prefer, swap the syrup for runny honey or agave nectar.

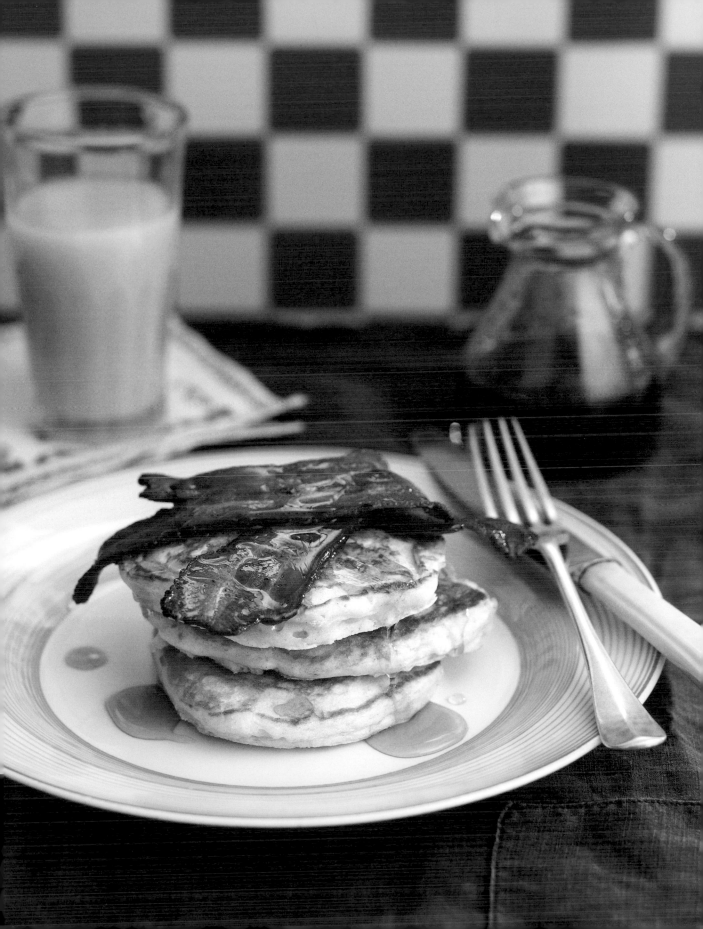

Smoky Beans on Toast

Once you've tried these, you may never go back to the tinned version (well, not as often!).

Hands-on time: 5 minutes
Cooking time: about
    25 minutes
Serves 6

1 tbsp olive oil
1 red onion, finely sliced
2 garlic cloves, crushed
2 tsp smoked paprika
3 x 400g tins mixed beans
   in water
2 tsp mustard powder
40g (1½oz) dark brown sugar
50g (2oz) tomato ketchup
200g (7oz) tomato passata
1½ tbsp white wine vinegar
Toast, to serve

PER SERVING 193cals,
9g protein, 3g fat (0g
saturates), 28g carbs (12g
total sugars), 9g fibre

1. In a large, deep frying pan or casserole, heat the oil over a medium heat. Add the onion, then cover with a lid and cook for 5 minutes. Stir in the garlic and paprika and fry for 1 minute until aromatic.

2. Add the beans (with their water) and the remaining ingredients. Bring to the boil, then bubble uncovered, stirring often, for 18–20 minutes until the sauce has reduced and thickened. Season the beans to taste with salt and pepper and serve on toast.

◆ GET AHEAD
Cool the beans after cooking and keep covered in the fridge for up to 3 days. To serve, reheat on the hob.

● GH TIP
Like traditional baked beans, these beans have a slight sweetness – if you prefer them less sweet, reduce the sugar to 25g (1oz).

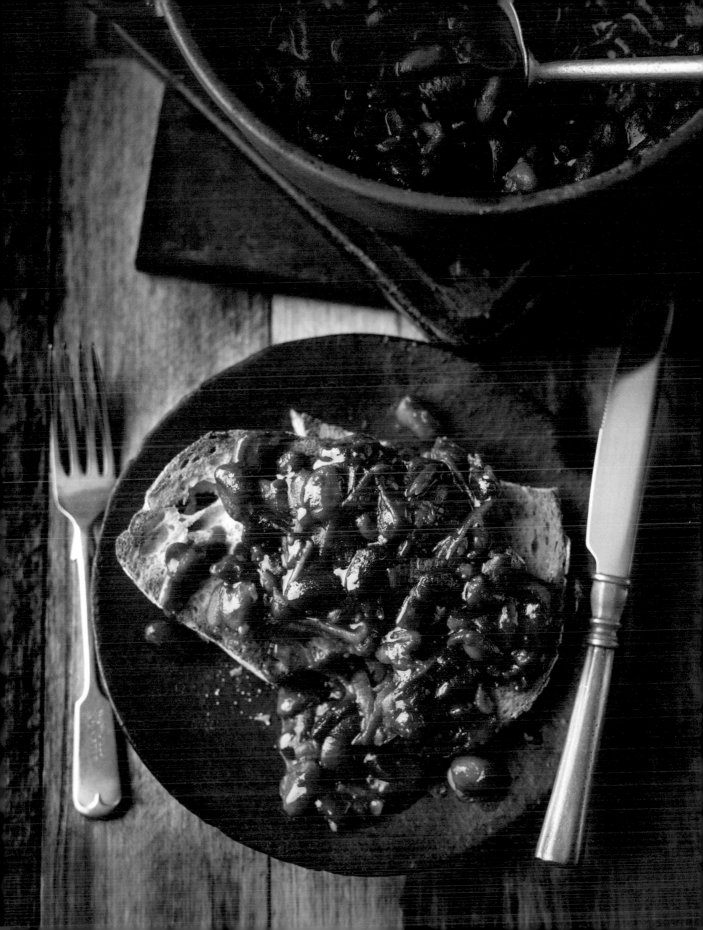

Smoked Haddock and Chorizo Omelette

Smoked fish and eggs are a classic brunch match, but adding a little chorizo gives them a bit of extra heat.

Hands-on time: 5 minutes
Cooking time: 5 minutes
Serves 4

25g (1oz) butter
2 shallots, finely sliced
100g (3½oz) chorizo ring, peeled and sliced
300g (11oz) skinless, undyed smoked haddock, cut into bite-size chunks
10 medium eggs, beaten
2 tbsp chopped fresh chives
Green salad, to serve (optional)

PER SERVING 369cals, 34g protein, 25g fat (9g saturates), 1g carbs (1g total sugars), 0.3g fibre

1. Heat the grill to medium-high. Put the butter in a 23cm (9in) ovenproof frying pan set over a high heat. Fry the shallots and chorizo for 1 minute, then add the haddock and fry, turning occasionally, for 1 minute to warm through.

2. Pour in the eggs. Season lightly, then scatter over the chives. Cook for 3 minutes on the hob, then transfer to the grill to cook the top until the egg is set and golden. Slide the omelette on to a board and serve in wedges with a crisp green salad.

Eggs Benedict

This brunch dish is a perennial favourite that never goes out of fashion.

Hands-on time: 25 minutes
Cooking time: about
    25 minutes
Serves 4

4 medium eggs
2 English muffins
4 ham slices
Cayenne pepper or chopped
   fresh chives, to serve
   (optional)

FOR THE HOLLANDAISE
SAUCE
2 medium egg yolks
1 tsp white wine vinegar
125g (4oz) unsalted butter,
   chilled and cubed

PER SERVING 454cals,
17g protein, 37g fat (20g
saturates), 16g carbs (1g
total sugars), 1g fibre

1. Bring a pan of lightly salted water to a simmer. Crack an egg into a coffee cup or ramekin. Swirl the water to create a whirlpool, then carefully tip in the egg. Repeat with a second egg. Simmer for 3–4 minutes until the whites are set but the yolks remain soft (lift an egg out with a slotted spoon and gently prod it to check). Transfer the cooked eggs to a shallow dish of warm water, then repeat with the remaining eggs.

2. While the second batch of eggs is cooking, split the muffins and toast them. Set them aside and keep warm.

3. To make the hollandaise, whisk the egg yolks and vinegar together in a small pan. Put the pan on a very gentle heat and whisk in a couple of cubes of butter until melted and combined. Then continue to whisk in the remaining butter, a couple of cubes at a time. Add a little water if the mixture seems too thick. Check the seasoning and remove from the heat.

4. Put a toasted muffin half on each of 4 plates, then lay a ham slice on top of each toasted muffin half. Lift the eggs out of the water, pat them dry, and put one on top of each muffin. Spoon some hollandaise over each egg and sprinkle over a little cayenne pepper or chopped chives (if using) and freshly ground black pepper. Serve.

● GH TIP
For Eggs Royale
Substitute slices of smoked salmon for the ham.

For Eggs Florentine
Replace the ham with wilted spinach for a veggie-friendly version.

Avocado and Poached Egg on Toast

A brunch classic. Mix up the spices, if you like – toasted cumin, fennel and coriander seeds or a pinch of lemony sumac make a nice change from chilli – or try swapping the lemon for lime juice.

Hands-on time: 10 minutes
Cooking time: 10 minutes
Serves 4

4 medium eggs
2 ripe avocados
Juice of 1 lemon
1 tsp chilli flakes or ½ red
  chilli, finely chopped
4 slices sourdough bread,
  toasted

PER SERVING 333cals,
12g protein, 21g fat (5g
saturates), 21g carbs (2g
total sugars), 5g fibre

1. Bring a pan of lightly salted water to a simmer. Crack an egg into a coffee cup or ramekin. Swirl the water to create a whirlpool, then carefully tip in the egg. Repeat with a second egg. Simmer for 3–4 minutes until the whites are set but the yolks remain soft (lift an egg out with a slotted spoon and gently prod it to check). Transfer the cooked eggs to a shallow dish of warm water, then repeat with the remaining eggs.

2. Meanwhile, halve and de-stone the avocados, then scoop out the flesh into a large bowl. Add the lemon juice and chilli and roughly mash. Season to taste.

3. Spread the avocado mixture over the toasted sourdough slices, top each slice with a poached egg and serve immediately.

◆ GET AHEAD
You can make the avocado mixture a few hours in advance and cover the surface with clingfilm – the lemon juice will help to keep it from turning brown.

How to Cook The Perfect Poached Eggs

The real secret is to use the freshest eggs you can find for poaching, as the egg whites are firmer and are less likely to spread out in the water. Add 1 teaspoon of white wine vinegar to the water, then bring it to the boil. Reduce the boiling water to a gentle simmer before adding the egg, as this will prevent the yolk from being too agitated and help to keep the egg white neat.

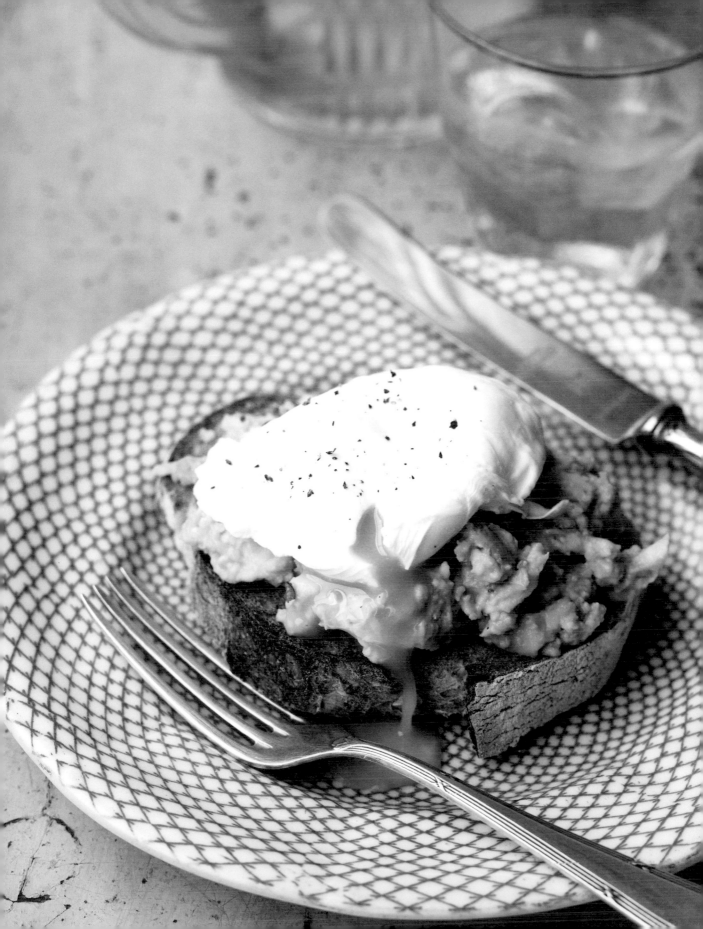

Mexican Bean Bowls

**This is a fun way to serve up a colourful, spicy salad.
The bean mixture also makes a tasty fajita filling.**

**Hands-on time: 20 minutes
Cooking time: 10 minutes
Serves 4**

2 tbsp olive oil
4 large flour tortillas
1 tsp smoked sweet paprika
1 small red onion, finely sliced
200g (7oz) cherry tomatoes,
    halved
2 avocados, peeled, stoned
    and chopped
400g tin mixed beans, drained
    and rinsed
400g tin kidney beans,
    drained and rinsed
198g tin sweetcorn, drained
Large bunch of fresh
    coriander, roughly chopped
4 large eggs, chilled

FOR THE DRESSING
2 tbsp red wine vinegar
½ tsp ground cumin
2 tbsp olive oil
1 tsp runny honey

**PER SERVING 593cals,
22g protein, 27g fat (6g
saturates), 58g carbs (11g
total sugars), 14g fibre**

1. Preheat the oven to 180°C (160°C fan) mark 4. Brush the oil over the tortillas, then sprinkle over a little paprika and some salt, and rub in. Flip over the tortillas and repeat on the opposite side. Loosely push each tortilla into its own small ovenproof bowl to bend it into a bowl shape, then cook the tortilla-filled bowls in the oven for 8–10 minutes until lightly golden and crisp. Cool the tortillas in the bowls to allow them to crisp up fully.

2. Meanwhile, bring a large pan of lightly salted water to the boil ready for poaching the eggs (see our top tips for perfectly poaching eggs on page 36).

3. Mix together the dressing ingredients in a large bowl. Then add the onion, tomatoes, avocados, both tins of beans, the sweetcorn and most of the coriander to the bowl and toss everything together. Check the seasoning and set aside.

4. Turn the boiling water down to a simmer. Crack an egg into a coffee cup or ramekin. Swirl the water to create a whirlpool, then carefully tip in the egg. Repeat with a second egg. Simmer for 3–4 minutes until the whites are set but the yolks remain soft (lift an egg out with a slotted spoon and gently prod it to check). Transfer the cooked eggs to a shallow dish of warm water, then repeat with the remaining eggs.

5. Remove the tortillas from their bowls. Divide the bean salad among the 4 tortilla bowls. Top each with a poached egg and sprinkle over the remaining coriander and some freshly ground black pepper.

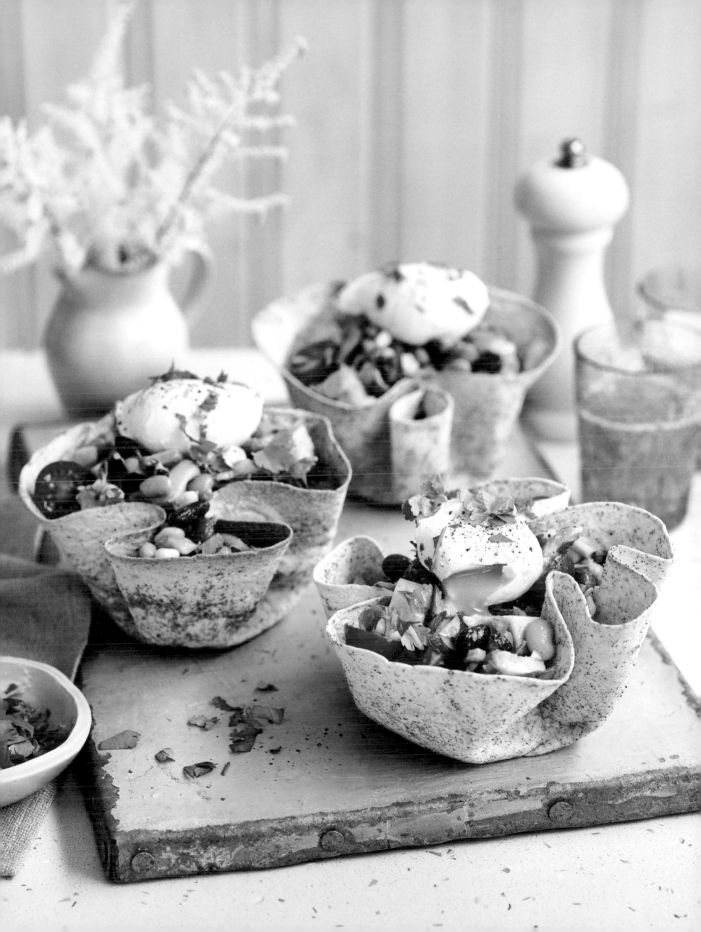

Crispy Crab Cakes

These cakes work equally well for brunch or supper, and can be made ahead of time if you're entertaining guests.

Hands-on time: 10 minutes
Cooking time: about
25 minutes
Serves 4

250g (9oz) white crab meat
4 spring onions, thinly sliced
7.5cm (3in) fresh root ginger,
   peeled and grated
4 tbsp fresh chives, finely
   chopped
1 red chilli, deseeded and
   finely chopped
2 large eggs
200g (7oz) fresh white
   breadcrumbs
3 tbsp vegetable oil
4 tbsp good-quality
   mayonnaise
Finely grated zest and juice
   of ½ lime, plus lime wedges
   to serve
Green salad, to serve
   (optional)

PER SERVING 398cals,
22g protein, 24g fat (2g
saturates), 24g carbs (2g
total sugars), 2g fibre

1. In a large bowl, mix together the crab, spring onions, ginger, chives, chilli, eggs and breadcrumbs. Season the mixture, then use your hands to form it into 16 round patties.

2. Heat the oil in a large non-stick frying pan. Working with a batch of 4 cakes at a time, fry the crab cakes for 6 minutes, turning once, until golden and crisp.

3. Meanwhile, mix together the mayonnaise, lime zest and juice. Season well and serve with the crab cakes, lime wedges and a crisp green salad, if you like.

◆ GET AHEAD
These crab cakes can be assembled up to 3 hours in advance. Once the cakes are made, cover them and chill. Bring back up to room temperature before cooking.

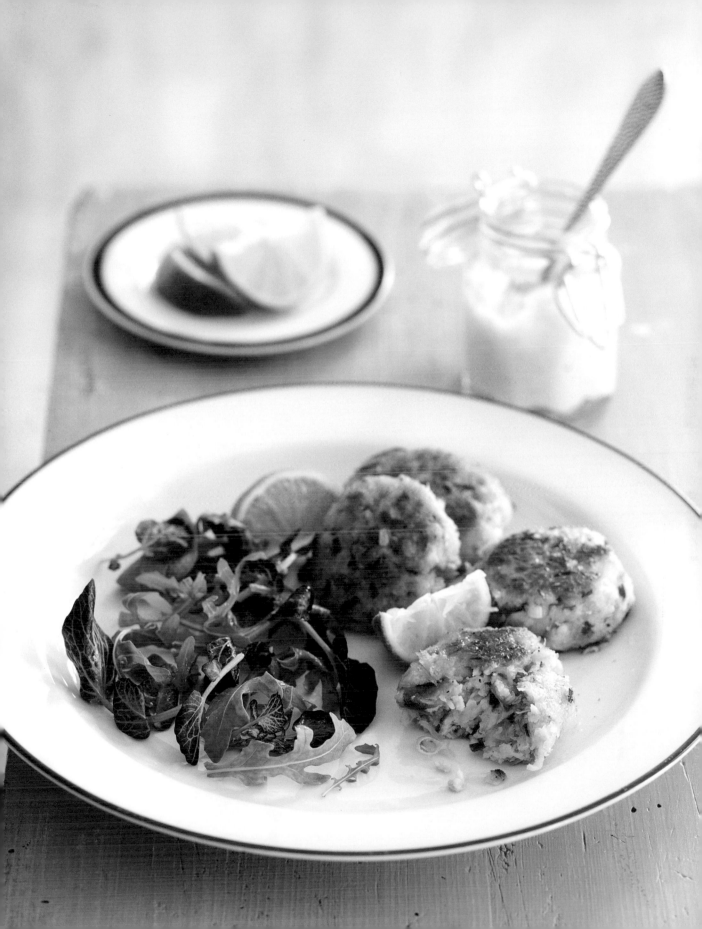

Halloumi and Pepper Bruschetta

The sweetness of these grilled peppers is an excellent match for salty halloumi. Grill some tomatoes with the peppers too, if you like.

Hands-on time: 5 minutes
Cooking time: about
   20 minutes
Serves 4

4 large mixed peppers,
   deseeded and sliced
2 tbsp extra virgin olive oil
250g pack halloumi, thinly
   sliced
8 slices sourdough bread
1 tbsp balsamic vinegar
Small handful of fresh mint,
   roughly chopped
Tzatziki or hummus, to serve

PER SERVING 475cals,
22g protein, 21g fat (11g
saturates), 46g carbs (9g
total sugars), 6g fibre

1. Heat the grill to medium. Put the pepper slices on a baking tray, drizzle over half of the oil and season well. Grill for 10–12 minutes, turning occasionally, until the peppers are tender and beginning to colour. Lay the halloumi slices over the peppers and grill for 5–6 minutes, turning once, until the cheese is golden.

2. When the halloumi is nearly ready, toast the bread. In a small bowl, stir together the remaining oil and balsamic vinegar with plenty of seasoning.

3. Divide the toasts, peppers and halloumi among 4 plates, then drizzle over the dressing. Scatter over the chopped mint and season with freshly ground black pepper. Serve immediately with a dollop of tzatziki or hummus.

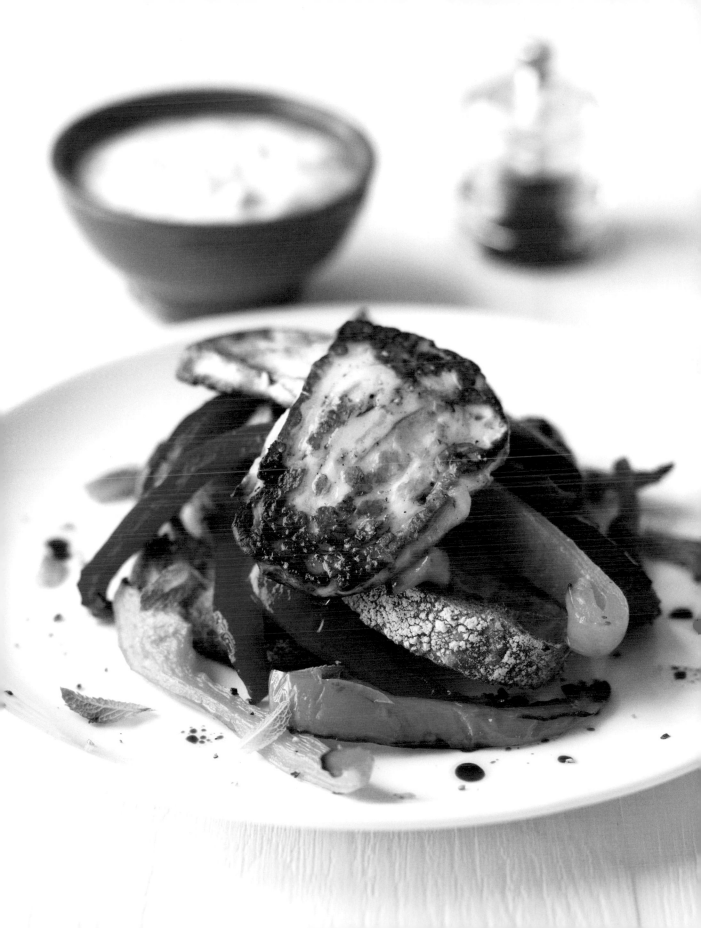

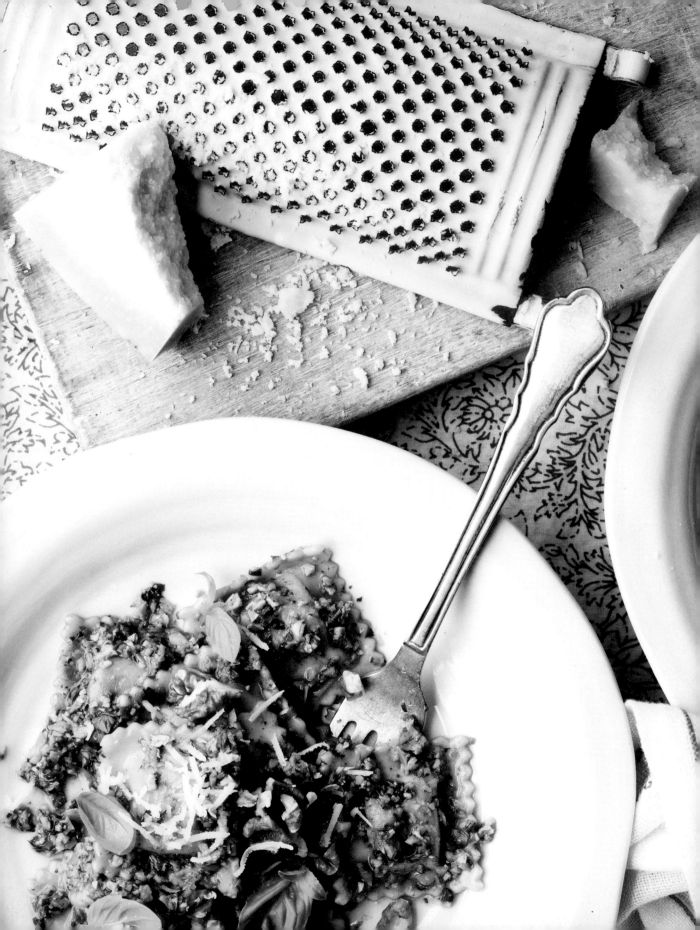

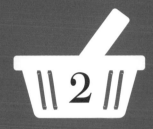

Take Five Ingredients

Creamy Chicken Chowder

Simple, hearty and warming, this soup truly is a meal in a bowl.

Hands-on time: 10 minutes
Cooking time: about
25 minutes
Serves 4

350g (12oz) chicken thigh
   fillets (skinless and
   boneless), cut into bite-size
   pieces
500g (1lb 2oz) potatoes,
   peeled and cut into 1cm
   (½in) pieces
750ml (1¼ pints) gluten-free
   chicken or vegetable stock
300g (11oz) frozen mixed
   vegetables
3–4 tbsp double cream, to
   taste

YOU WILL ALSO NEED
1 tbsp olive oil

PER SERVING 361cals,
22g protein, 18g fat (6g
saturates), 26g carbs (4g
total sugars), 3g fibre

1. Heat the oil in a large frying pan. Add the chicken pieces and cook over a high heat for 5–10 minutes, stirring until golden. Remove the pan from the heat and transfer the chicken to a plate.

2. Meanwhile, add the potatoes to another pan and pour over the stock. Bring to the boil and simmer for 10–15 minutes until the potatoes are completely tender. Remove a spoonful of the potatoes and mash them to a purée, then return this to the pan to help thicken the broth. Add the chicken and simmer for 5 minutes until the chicken is cooked through.

3. Add the vegetables and cream. Bring back up to the boil, then reduce the heat and simmer for a few minutes. Season to taste. Ladle the soup into deep bowls and serve with a fresh grinding of black pepper.

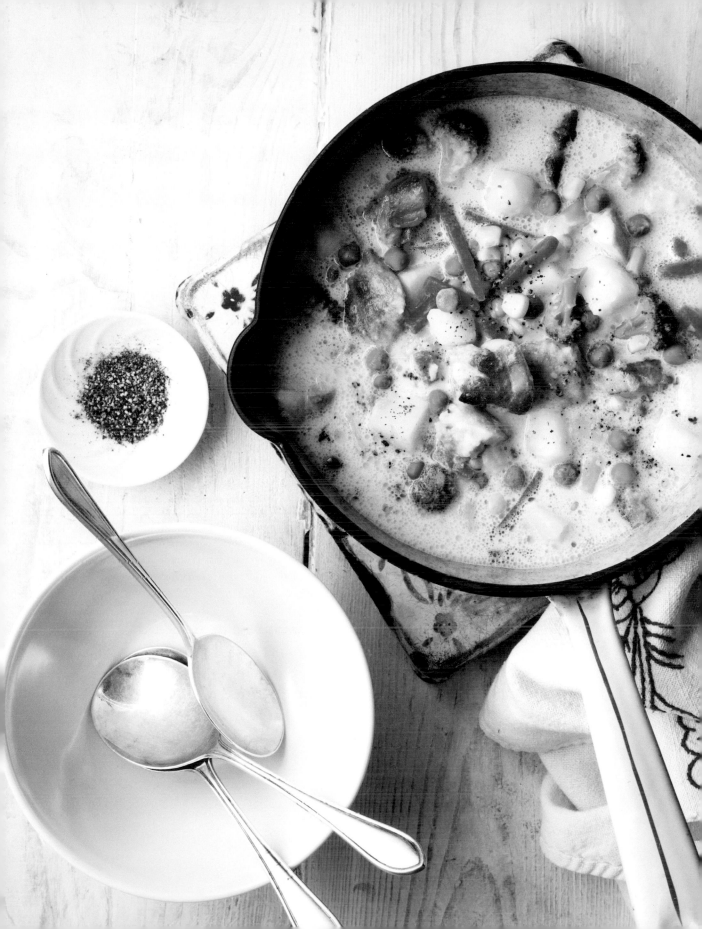

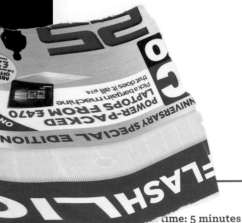

Bloody Mary Tortelloni Soup

Adding filled pasta to a ready-made soup transforms it from a light lunch to a more substantial meal, and you can easily adapt it to suit meat-eaters or vegetarians.

time: 5 minutes
Cooking time: about
   10 minutes
Serves 4

3 x 600g tubs fresh tomato
   and basil soup
Zest and juice of 1 lemon
¼–½ tsp Tabasco sauce, to
   taste
50ml (2fl oz) vodka, optional
300g (11oz) tortelloni or
   ravioli in your favourite
   flavour

PER SERVING 313cals,
9g protein, 9g fat (2g
saturates), 41g carbs (23g
total sugars), 5g fibre

1. In a large pan, gently heat the soup until it's piping hot. Add the lemon zest and juice, Tabasco and the vodka, if using. Season with plenty of black pepper.

2. Add the pasta and cook in the soup until tender – about 1–2 minutes. Divide among 4 warm soup bowls and serve.

Carbonara

This timeless recipe is often made with cream in restaurants, but we've gone authentic and used the pasta cooking water for a lighter and more traditional version.

Hands-on time: 10 minutes
Cooking time: about
   15 minutes
Serves 4

350g (12oz) dried linguine
200g (7oz) unsmoked bacon
   lardons or cubed pancetta
4 large eggs, beaten
75g (3oz) Parmesan, grated,
   plus extra to serve
Handful of fresh flat-leaf
   parsley, chopped

YOU WILL ALSO NEED
½ tbsp olive oil

PER SERVING 622cals,
32g protein, 26g fat (10g
saturates), 63g carbs (2g
total sugars), 4g fibre

1. Bring a large pan of salted water to the boil and cook the pasta according to the pack instructions. Meanwhile, put the olive oil in a large frying pan set over a medium heat. Fry the bacon lardons for 5 minutes or until golden, then take the pan off the heat.

2. In a medium bowl, mix together the beaten eggs, grated Parmesan and plenty of freshly ground black pepper. Drain the pasta, reserving 100ml (3½fl oz) of the cooking water.

3. Return the bacon pan to a very low heat and stir in the pasta water, cooked pasta and the egg mixture, tossing with tongs for about 1 minute until the sauce begins to thicken and coat the pasta.

4. Check the seasoning, then divide the pasta among 4 bowls or plates. Sprinkle with chopped fresh parsley and extra Parmesan and serve.

Fig, Blue Cheese and Pesto Tart

This tart is easy to assemble, and you can vary the flavour by using a different type of pesto. Add some cubed pancetta to the uncooked tart if you fancy making it meaty.

Hands-on time: 10 minutes
Cooking time: about
   20 minutes
Serves 4

320g sheet ready rolled
   puff pastry
4 tbsp fresh basil pesto
3 fresh figs, quartered
75g (3oz) vegetarian blue
   cheese, we used Stilton
Handful of rocket leaves, plus
   extra to serve

PER SERVING 526cals,
14g protein, 40g fat (15g
saturates), 27g carbs (4g
total sugars), 2g fibre

1. Preheat the oven to 200°C (180°C fan) mark 6. Unroll the pastry on to a baking sheet, leaving it on the baking paper it comes on. Score a border 2.5cm (1in) in from the edge all the way around with a knife (taking care not to cut right through the pastry). Prick the pastry well with a fork inside the border.

2. Spread the pesto in an even layer inside the border, then scatter over the figs. Crumble the blue cheese evenly over the surface. Bake for 20 minutes or until the pastry is risen, golden and cooked through.

3. Scatter over the rocket and serve the tart in quarters with extra rocket on the side, if you like.

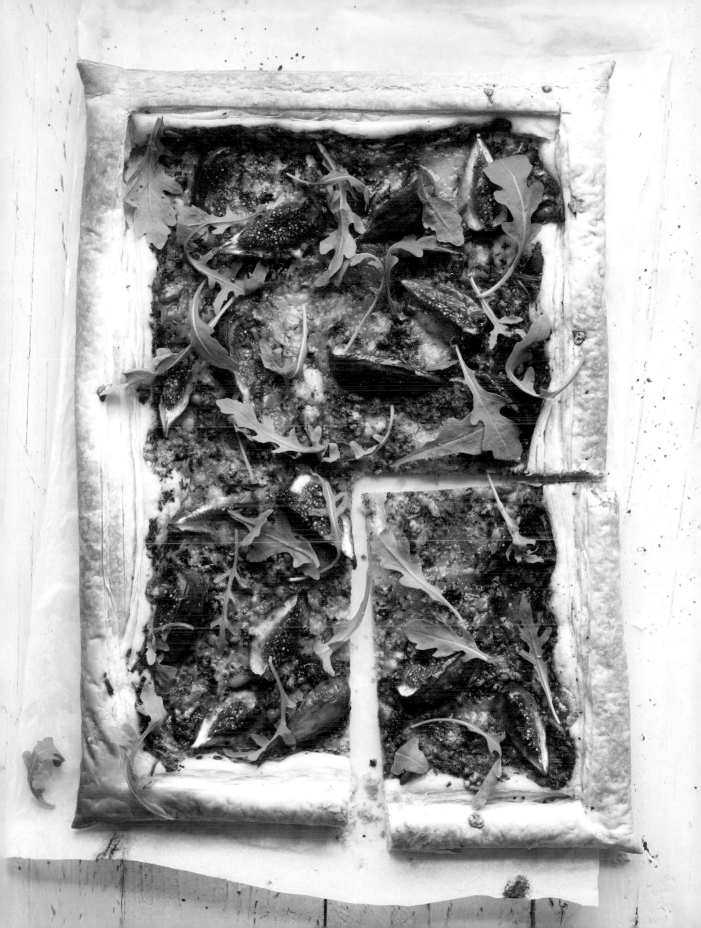

Artichoke Pesto Ravioli

A super-speedy vegetarian supper with a great mix of flavours.

Hands-on time: 10 minutes
Cooking time: about
5 minutes
Serves 4

50g (2oz) basil, including
   stalks
150g (5oz) chargrilled
   artichokes from a jar
   (reserve the oil)
50g (2oz) walnut halves
50g (2oz) Parmesan cheese
   or vegetarian alternative,
   coarsely grated, plus extra
   to serve
About 600g (1lb 5oz) spinach
   and ricotta ravioli or
   tortellini

YOU WILL ALSO NEED
Extra virgin olive oil

PER SERVING 492cals,
17g protein, 29g fat (8g
saturates), 38g carbs (3g
total sugars), 7g fibre

1. Reserve a few basil leaves to use as garnish, then put the remaining basil into a food processor (stalks and all) with the artichokes, about 4 tablespoons oil (made up of reserved artichoke oil and olive oil, if needed), most of the walnuts, the Parmesan and some seasoning. Whiz to a chunky, pesto-like consistency.

2. Bring a large pan of water to the boil and cook the pasta according to the pack instructions.

3. Drain the cooked pasta, reserving a cupful of the cooking water. Put the pesto into the empty pan and return it to a low heat, adding enough of the reserved water to loosen. Add the cooked pasta and toss gently to coat. To serve, divide the pasta among 4 bowls. Top each portion with the remaining walnuts, basil leaves and grated Parmesan.

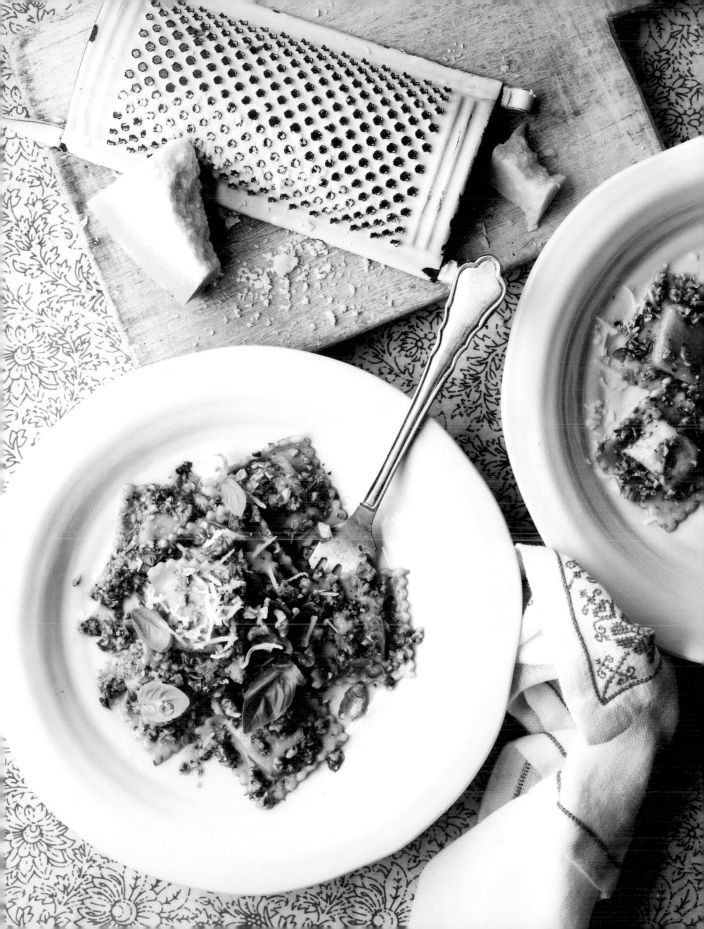

Pasta con le Sarde

Raid the storecupboard for our take on this traditional Sicilian dish, which combines spaghetti with fish.

Hands-on time: 10 minutes
Cooking time: about
   15 minutes
Serves 4

75g (3oz) pinenuts
1 large bulb fennel
2 x 120g tins sardines in oil
350g (12oz) spaghetti
75g (3oz) mixed vine fruit
   or raisins
Lemon wedges, to squeeze
   over

**PER SERVING 614cals,
26g protein, 21g fat (3g
saturates), 77g carbs (16g
total sugars), 8g fibre**

1. Add the pinenuts to a dry non-stick frying pan and cook over a medium heat for 2–3 minutes, shaking the pan occasionally until the nuts are toasted. Tip into a bowl to cool slightly.

2. Slice the delicate fronds off the fennel and set them aside to use as a garnish, then finely chop the remaining fennel bulb. Drain the oil from 1 tin of sardines into the frying pan. Add the chopped fennel and fry for 5 minutes until just beginning to soften.

3. Meanwhile, in a large pan of salted boiling water, cook the pasta according to the pack instructions.

4. Add the sardines from the drained tin to the frying pan, along with the mixed vine fruit or raisins and 200ml (7fl oz) water. Stir to break up the sardines, then season and simmer for 5 minutes.

5. Drain the pasta, return it to the empty pan and pour over the sauce along with the remaining sardines, drained (discard the oil). Toss the pasta with tongs to distribute the sauce. Season to taste and divide among 4 bowls. Sprinkle over the reserved fennel fronds and pinenuts. Serve with lemon wedges to squeeze over, if you like.

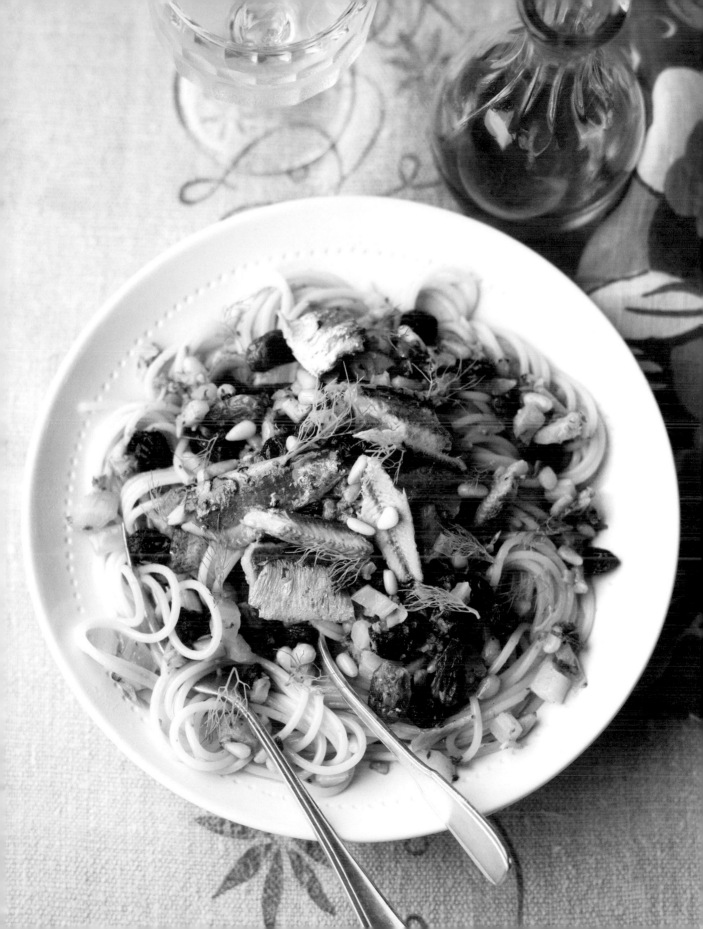

Jamaican-style Prawn Pepper Pot

Jerk spice mix is a Jamaican-style spice blend. Aromatic and hot, it combines chilli with other piquant flavours such as cinnamon, nutmeg and garlic, and is a mainstay of Caribbean cooking.

Hands-on time: 5 minutes
Cooking time: about
   10 minutes
Serves 4

3 mixed peppers, deseeded
   and chopped
1 tbsp gluten-free jerk
   spice mix
2 x 235g packs frozen raw
   prawns, defrosted (excess
   liquid drained away)
Zest and juice of 1 lemon
100ml (3fl oz) gluten-free
   chicken stock

YOU WILL ALSO NEED
1 tbsp olive oil

PER SERVING 162cals,
24g protein, 4g fat (1g
saturates), 7g carbs (7g total
sugars), 2g fibre

1. Heat the oil in a large frying pan over a high heat and fry the peppers for 5 minutes until softened and slightly charred.

2. Stir in the jerk spice mix and cook for 1 minute, then add the prawns, lemon zest and juice, and stock. Cook until all the prawns are pink. Check the seasoning and serve with rice, if you like.

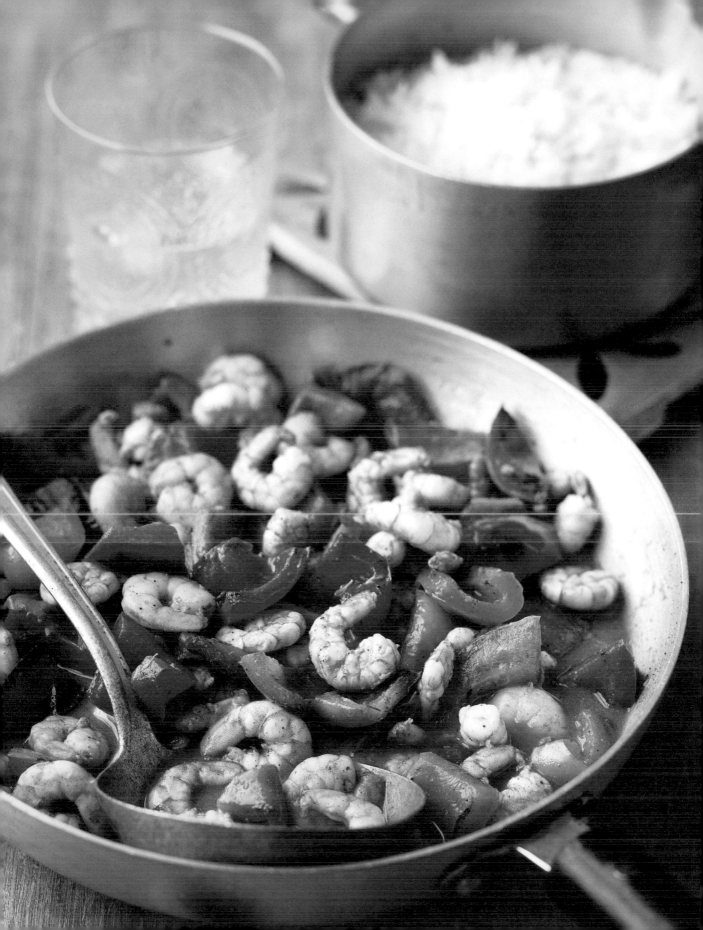

Gnocchi and Chorizo Gratin

If you're a fan of mac 'n' cheese, this one's for you! There's no need to boil the gnocchi, so it's ready in a flash.

Hands-on time: 15 minutes
**Cooking time: about
    15 minutes**
Serves 4

125g (4oz) cooking chorizo
    sausages, quartered
1kg (2lb 3½oz) fresh gnocchi
250g (9oz) full-fat cream
    cheese
125g (4oz) frozen peas,
    defrosted
50g (2oz) mature Cheddar,
    grated

**PER SERVING 893cals,
24g protein, 43g fat (24g
saturates), 101g carbs (2g
total sugars), 5g fibre**

1. Heat the grill to medium–high. Meanwhile, set a large frying pan over a medium heat and fry the chorizo until golden and crisp. Remove with a slotted spoon to a plate, then return the pan to the heat. Add the gnocchi in batches and fry in the chorizo oil for 2–3 minutes, tossing the pan occasionally, until the gnocchi is golden. Add to the plate with the chorizo.

2. Add the cream cheese to the pan along with 125ml (4fl oz) just-boiled water. Stir to combine and heat through, then season with freshly ground black pepper. Stir in the peas. Return the gnocchi and chorizo to the pan and mix well. Tip into a 2 litre (3½ pint) ovenproof baking dish and scatter over the Cheddar cheese. Grill for 4–5 minutes until bubbling and golden, then serve.

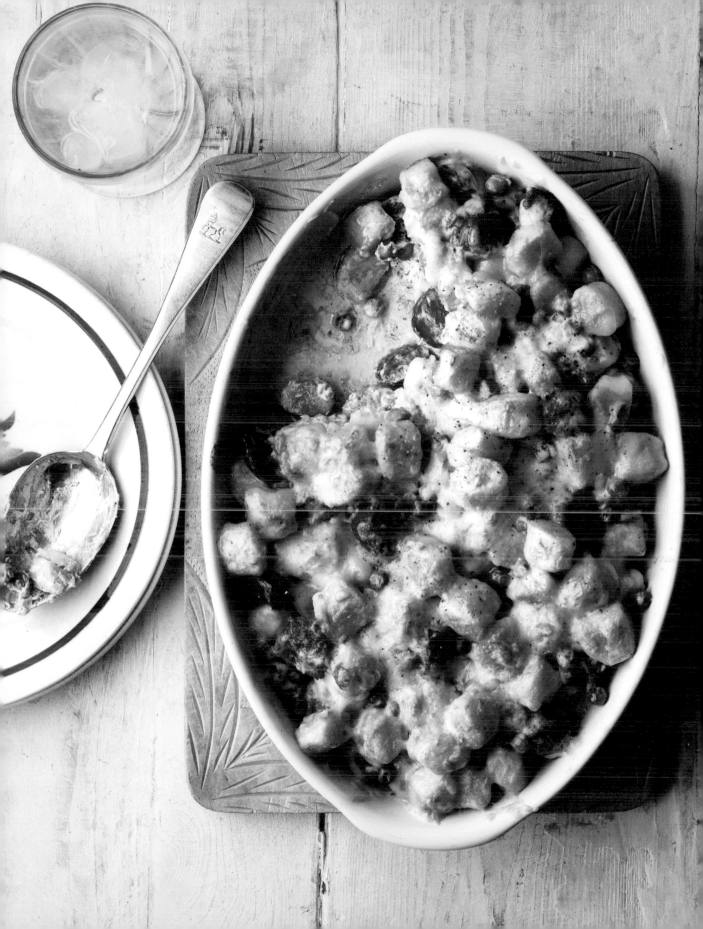

Herby Chicken and Cannellini Bean Stew

Light, fresh and high in fibre, this simple family supper is great on its own, or serve it with fresh crusty bread to mop up the juices, if it doesn't need to be gluten free. A good quality chicken stock will make all the difference here.

Hands-on time: 15 minutes
Cooking time: about
    15 minutes
Serves 4

4 skinless chicken breasts
3 x 400g tins cannellini beans,
    drained and rinsed
750ml (1¼ pints) gluten-free
    chicken stock
Finely grated zest of 1 lemon
25g pack fresh parsley,
    roughly chopped (including
    stalks)

YOU WILL ALSO NEED
2 tbsp extra virgin olive oil

**PER SERVING 328cals,
45g protein, 7g fat (1g
saturates), 16g carbs (2g
total sugars), 8g fibre**

1. Slice the chicken into finger-size strips. Heat the olive oil in a large pan and fry the chicken for a couple of minutes to start it cooking.

2. Add the beans, stock and some seasoning to the pan. Bring to the boil, then simmer for 10 minutes or until the chicken is cooked through.

3. Stir in the lemon zest and parsley. Check the seasoning. Ladle into bowls, drizzle over a little extra oil and serve.

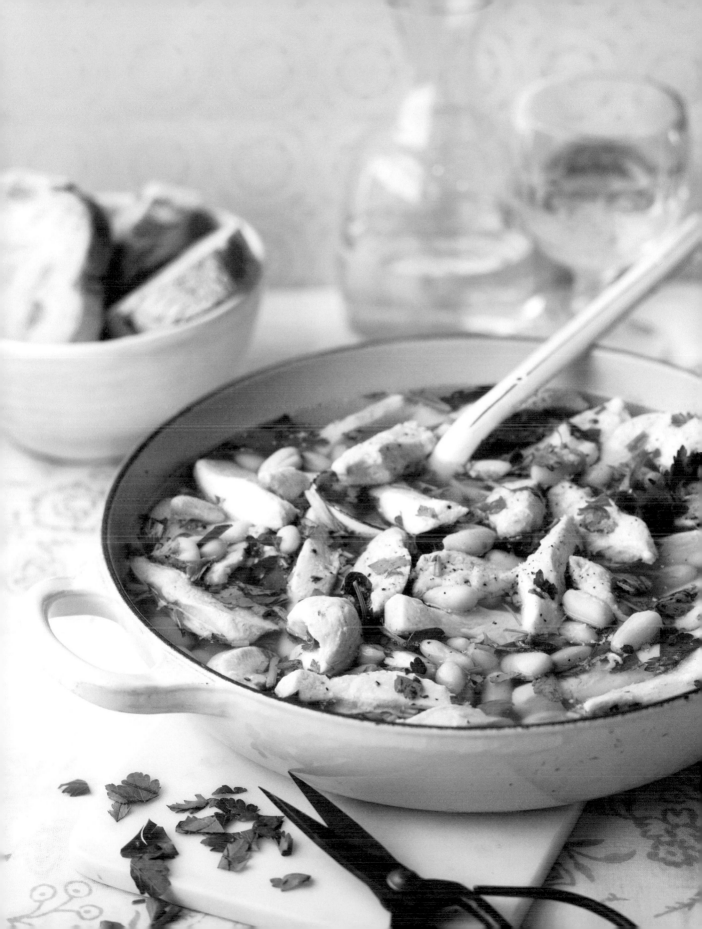

Prawn and Spinach Curry

We've spiced up ready-made soup with some curry paste for a super quick, simple curry that's ready in minutes. Delicious for a light lunch as it is, or serve it with rice or naan breads (if it doesn't need to be gluten free) for a more filling meal.

Hands-on time: 10 minutes
Cooking time: about
   10 minutes
Serves 4

1½ tbsp gluten-free mild
   curry paste
2 x 600g tubs thick red lentil
   and tomato soup
300g (11oz) frozen cooked and
   peeled king prawns
100g bag baby spinach

**PER SERVING 172cals,
21g protein, 4g fat (0.4g
saturates), 12g carbs (6g
total sugars), 4g fibre**

1. Set a large non-stick pan over a medium heat. Stir-fry the curry paste for about 30 seconds until fragrant to wake up the flavours. Add the soup, bring to the boil and simmer for 5 minutes until it reaches the desired thickness for your sauce.

2. Add the prawns and simmer for a couple of minutes to heat them through, then stir in the spinach. Check the seasoning and serve as it is, or with rice or naans (if it doesn't need to be gluten free) to mop up the juices.

● GH TIP
For special diets, check the labels on your soup and curry paste. Both should be dairy free, and many options will be gluten free, too.

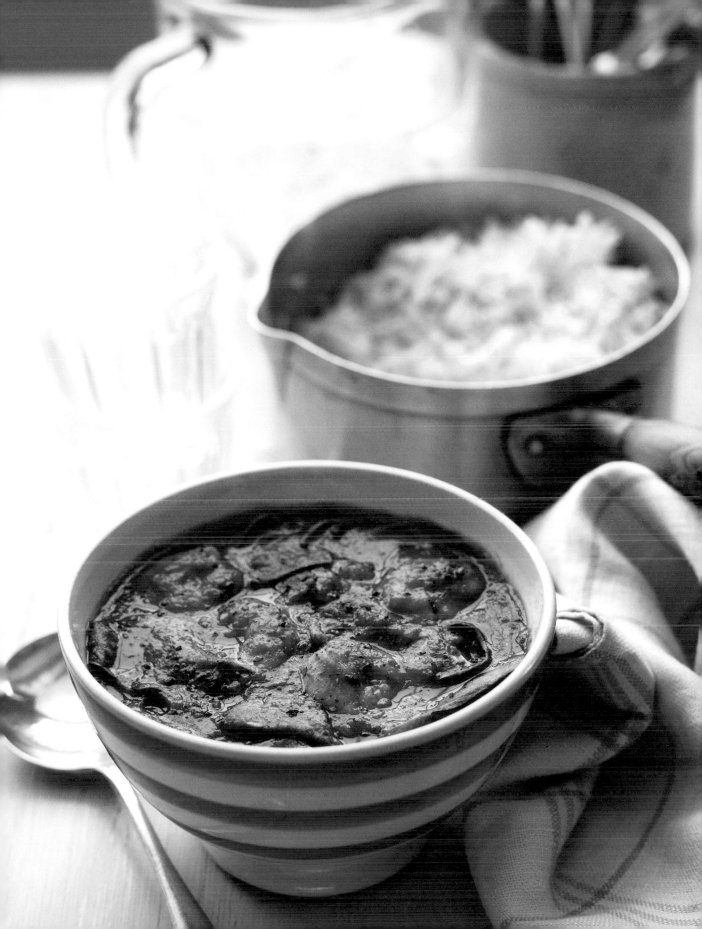

Hoisin Beef

A great choice for a weeknight supper, this speedy dish will also boost your five-a-day. The vegetables are stir-fried quickly, so make sure your beef is sliced before you begin cooking.

Hands-on time: 15 minutes
Cooking time: about
  10 minutes
Serves 4

3 x 300g packs stir-fry
   vegetable mix
225g (8oz) dried instant
   rice noodles
3 rump steaks, fat trimmed,
   sliced into strips 1cm
   (½in) wide
3 tbsp hoisin sauce
2 tbsp sesame seeds

YOU WILL ALSO NEED
2 tbsp vegetable oil

**PER SERVING 559cals,
41g protein, 16g fat (4g
saturates), 60g carbs (12g
total sugars), 5g fibre**

1. Put 1 tablespoon of the oil in a large wok or frying pan set over a high heat. Add the vegetables, season well, and stir-fry for 3–5 minutes until tender.

2. Meanwhile, put the noodles in a large heatproof bowl and cover with freshly boiled water from the kettle. Set aside for 3 minutes to soak, then drain.

3. Tip the cooked noodles on to a serving platter and top with the vegetables. Cover with foil to keep warm.

4. Return the wok/frying pan to high heat and add the remaining tablespoon of oil. Fry the steak strips for 1 minute, then add the hoisin sauce and 50ml (2fl oz) water. Simmer for 30 seconds, then remove from the heat and spoon the steak and sauce over the vegetables. Scatter over the sesame seeds and serve.

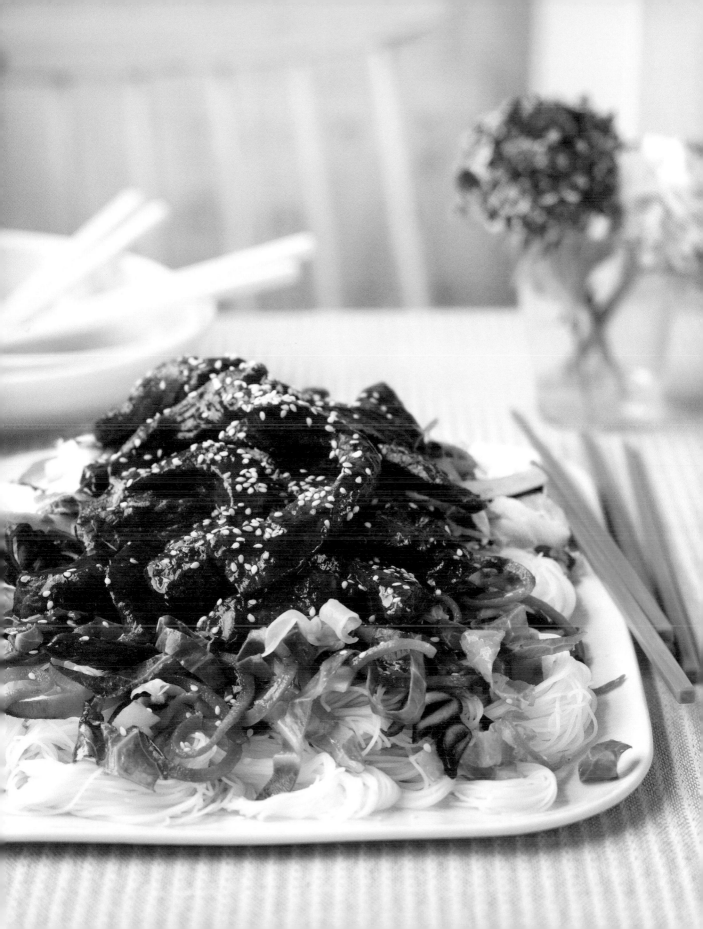

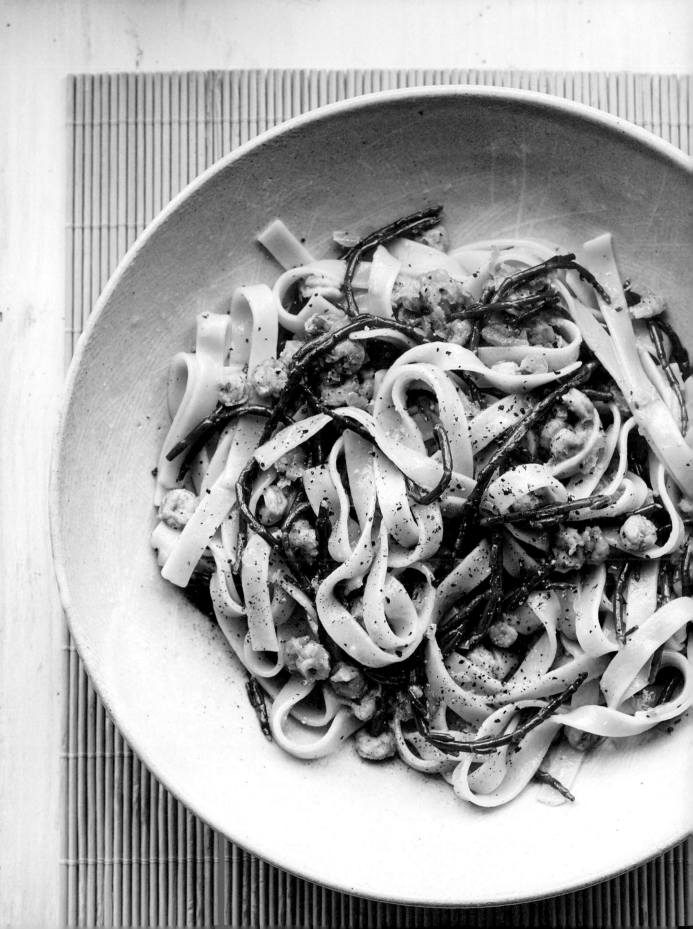

3

Cooking for One

Cooking for one – top tips

• Don't be afraid to make big batches or a roast – simply plan meals around leftovers or use ingredients that freeze well.

• Stock your storecupboard with flavourful ingredients. Coconut cream, fish sauce, soy sauce, sriracha, pomegranate molasses, Marmite, balsamic vinegar and Worcestershire sauce will transform simple meals.

• Instead of buying packets of herbs that may wilt before you've used them up, choose living pots.

• Make the most of your freezer: grated cheese, nuts, chopped soft herbs in oil, wine ice cubes and pesto are freezer-friendly standbys that make great flavour enhancers. Just label items clearly with a date.

• Shop at the meat/fish/deli counters in store rather than buying pre-packaged items – you can buy a single salmon fillet or just the right amount of cheese you need, and you'll help to cut your food costs and reduce waste.

• If scaling down recipes, remember that spices, herbs and seasonings may not need reducing as much as bulky ingredients such as meat and veg. Add condiments to taste.

• Baking needn't be off limits. Lots of biscuits can be frozen before or after baking, and many cakes freeze well when sliced (a perfect solution for controlling portions). Aim to freeze cakes that don't have icing (although cream cheese icings do freeze well).

Cheese and Watercress Omelette

Omelettes are so versatile, and a great way to use up your favourite ingredients or leftovers. You can always add an extra egg if you're particularly hungry.

Hands-on time: 5 minutes
Cooking time: about
** 2–3 minutes**
Serves 1

½ tbsp vegetable oil
2 large eggs, lightly beaten
Small handful of watercress,
    roughly chopped
25g (1oz) Gruyère-style
    vegetarian cheese

PER SERVING 320cals,
23g protein, 25g fat (9g
saturates), 0g carbs (0g
total sugars), 1g fibre

1. Put the oil in a small frying pan set over a high heat. Season the eggs and add to the pan. When the egg begins to set at the edges of the pan, use a spatula to draw the set egg into the centre, tilting the pan if you need to to allow runny egg to spread into the gaps.

2. After a few minutes, when the top of the omelette is almost fully set, add the chopped watercress and cheese. When the base of the omelette is golden (use the spatula to carefully lift the omelette and check it) and the cheese is melting, fold it in half and transfer to a plate. Serve the omelette with a green salad and some gluten-free bread, if you like.

● GH TIP
You can easily vary the omelette fillings to suit your diet or what you have available. Next time, try adding smoked salmon pieces and a handful of peppery rocket.

TOAST TOPPERS

These slices make a great breakfast, brunch or lunch and you'll soon be creating your own flavour combinations.

Goat's Cheese and Fig on Toast

Hands-on time: 15 minutes
Serves 1

PER SERVING 233cals, 10g protein, 11g fat (7g saturates), 22g carbs (4g total sugars), 2g fibre

2 tbsp goat's cheese
1 tbsp soured cream
Pinch of fresh or dried thyme leaves
1 slice bread, toasted
1 fig, quartered
Honey, to drizzle
Walnuts, toasted, to serve

1. In a small bowl, whisk together the goat's cheese, soured cream and thyme leaves with plenty of freshly ground black pepper.

2. Spread the mixture over the toast and top with a quartered fig, a drizzle of honey and a sprinkle of toasted walnuts.

Beetroot, Avocado and Feta Cheese on Toast

Hands-on time: 5 minutes
Serves 1

PER SERVING 372cals, 10g protein, 26g fat (9g saturates), 23g carbs (3g total sugars), 5g fibre

1 slice bread, toasted
2 tbsp beetroot dip or hummus
½ avocado, sliced
25g (1oz) vegetarian feta, crumbled
A few pomegranate seeds, to serve
Olive oil, to drizzle

1. Spread the toast with the beetroot dip or hummus, then top with the sliced avocado, crumbled feta and a sprinkle of pomegranate seeds. Drizzle over a little olive oil and serve.

Spicy Egg and Asparagus on Toast

Hands-on time: 5 minutes
Cooking time: 10 minutes
Serves 1

PER SERVING 260cals, 14g protein, 13g fat (5g saturates), 21g carbs (2g total sugars), 3g fibre

1 large egg
Small handful of asparagus spears, trimmed
1 slice bread, toasted
½ tsp butter, to spread
Sriracha sauce, to serve
Mixed seeds, to sprinkle

1. Cook the egg in simmering water for 7 minutes. Drain and cool under cold running water, then peel the egg and slice in half.

2. Meanwhile, cook the asparagus spears in a pan of boiling water for 3 minutes. Drain well.

3. Spread a slice of toast with the butter and top with the asparagus spears and egg halves. Drizzle over a little sriracha sauce and sprinkle with mixed seeds.

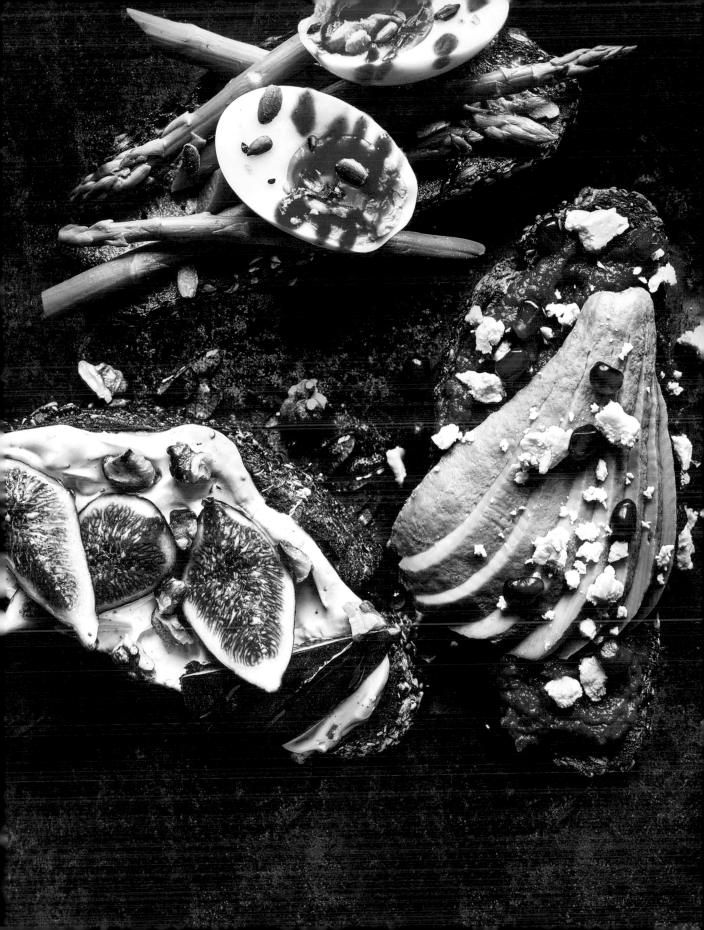

Steak Sandwich

Planning a quiet night in? This hearty sandwich is easy and delicious, yet still filling enough to enjoy as an evening meal.

Hands-on time: 10 minutes, plus resting
Cooking time: about 6 minutes
Serves 1

200g (7oz) rump steak
1 tbsp extra virgin olive oil, plus extra to drizzle (optional)
Ciabatta bread roll
Small handful of rocket or spinach
Parmesan, shaved, or blue cheese, crumbled, to serve (optional)

PER SERVING (without cheese or extra oil) 496cals, 51g protein, 21g fat (5g saturates), 25g carbs (2g total sugars), 2g fibre

1. Pat the steak dry with kitchen paper and season well. Put the oil in a frying pan set over a high heat, then fry the steak for 2–3 minutes on each side for medium (cook the steak for shorter or longer, if you prefer). Transfer the cooked steak to a board, cover with foil and leave to rest for 5 minutes.

2. Meanwhile, slice the bread roll in half horizontally. Toast the halves, cut-sides down, in the empty steak pan for 1 minute. Remove from the heat.

3. Use a serrated knife to slice the steak. Put the toasted bottom half of the roll on a plate, then top it with the steak slices and a handful of rocket or spinach leaves. Add some shaved Parmesan or crumbled blue cheese and drizzle over a little extra virgin olive oil, if you like. Sandwich together with the top of the roll and serve.

● GH TIP
Next time, try swapping the steak for a cooked salmon fillet, roughly flaked, with a handful of rocket and some tartar sauce.

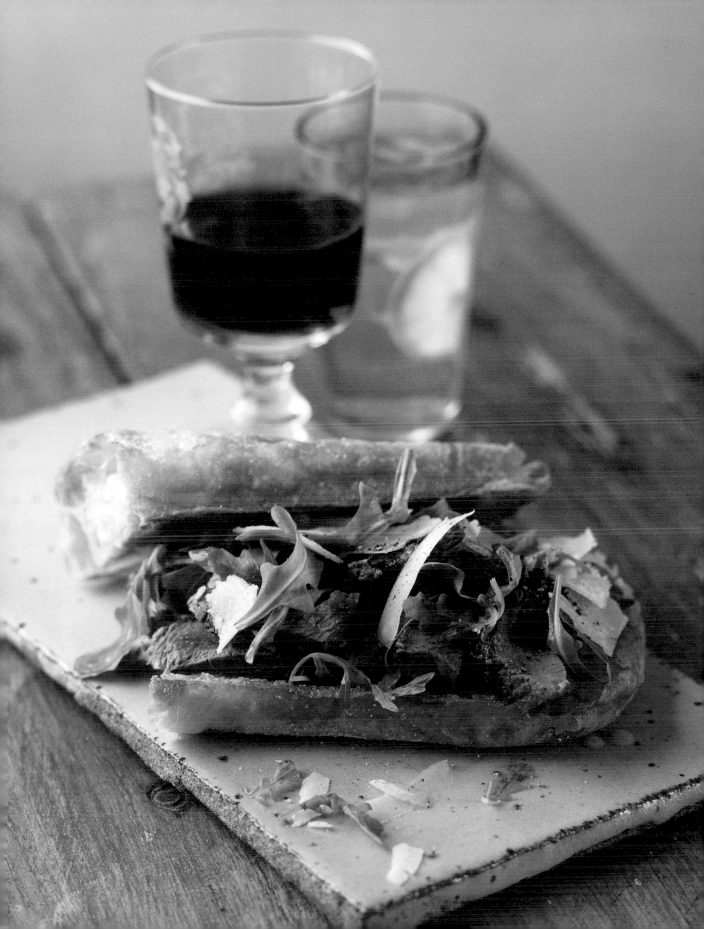

SCANDI-STYLE OPEN SANDWICHES

A favourite in Nordic countries, these rye bread sandwiches make a speedy light lunch or quick summer supper.

Ricotta, Radish and Egg

Hands-on time: 5 minutes
Cooking time: 10 minutes
Makes 1 sandwich

PER SERVING 240cals, 15g protein, 10g fat (5g saturates), 20g carbs (4g total sugars), 4g fibre

1 large egg
Spray oil
4 asparagus spears
2 tbsp vegetarian ricotta
1 slice rye bread
2 radishes, sliced

1. Cook the egg in simmering water for 9 minutes. Drain and cool under cold running water, then peel the egg and slice in half. (Save one of the halves in the fridge to use for another sandwich.)

2. Meanwhile, spray a small griddle pan with oil and set over a medium heat. Griddle the asparagus spears for 3 minutes, turning once.

3. Spread the ricotta on a slice of rye bread. Top with the griddled asparagus, half a hard-boiled egg and the radish slices. Serve.

Avo and Hot-smoked Salmon

Hand-on time: 5 minutes
Makes 1 sandwich

PER SERVING 349cals, 12g protein, 24g fat (8g saturates), 20g carbs (2g total sugars), 6g fibre

½ avocado, mashed
1 slice rye bread
25g (1oz) hot-smoked salmon
1 tbsp crème fraîche
1 tsp capers
Fresh dill, to garnish

1. Spread the avocado on a slice of rye bread. Top with the flaked salmon, followed by a dollop of crème fraîche, the capers and a sprinkling of dill. Serve.

Ham and Artichokes

Hands-on time: 5 minutes
Makes 1 sandwich

PER SERVING 219cals, 8g protein, 11g fat (2g saturates), 19g carbs (1g total sugars), 5g fibre

1 tbsp basil pesto
1 slice rye bread
1 slice Parma ham
2 artichokes from a jar, drained and sliced
A few rocket leaves, to garnish

1. Spread the pesto on a slice of rye bread. Top with the slice of ham, the artichoke slices and a few rocket leaves and serve immediately.

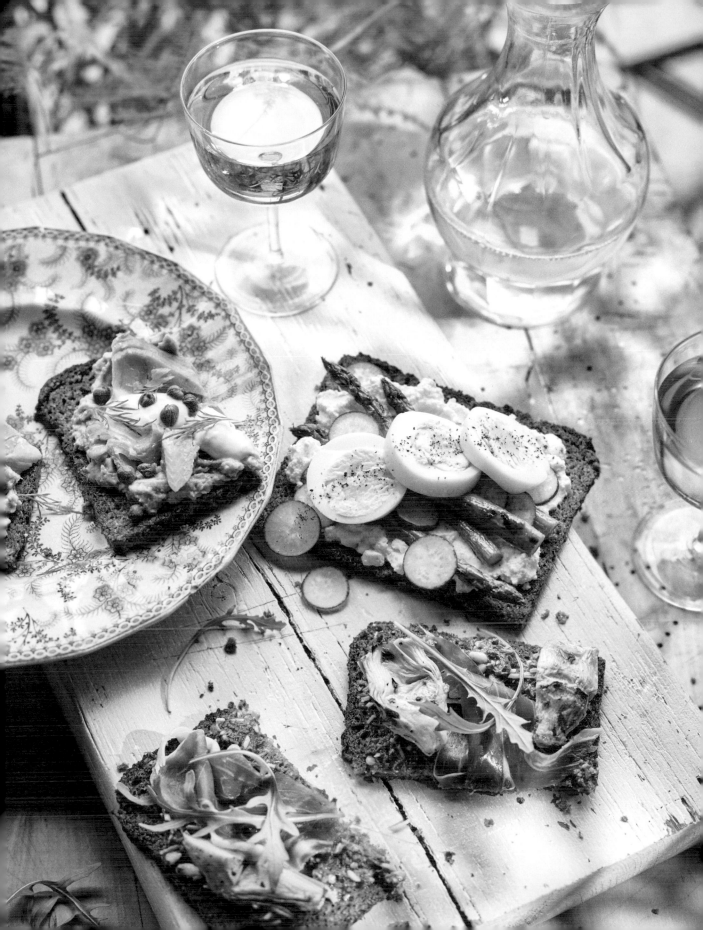

Courgette, Mint and Goat's Cheese Fritters with Tzatziki

These flavoursome fritters are easy to whip up. Swap the goat's cheese for feta, if you prefer.

Hands-on time: 20 minutes, plus salting
Cooking time: about 10 minutes
Serves 1

150g (5oz) courgettes (roughly 2 small courgettes)
½ lemon
40g (1½oz) self-raising flour
1 medium egg, beaten
40g (1½oz) soft vegetarian goat's cheese, crumbled
2 tbsp chopped fresh mint
2 spring onions, finely chopped
2 tbsp olive oil

FOR THE TZATZIKI
60g (2½oz) Greek yogurt
¼ cucumber, deseeded and finely diced
1 small garlic clove, crushed
1 tbsp chopped fresh mint

PER SERVING 642cals, 28g protein, 42g fat (14g saturates), 37g carbs (7g total sugars), 4g fibre

1. Coarsely grate the courgettes and put into a sieve set over a bowl. Sprinkle with a couple of pinches of salt and let sit for 20 minutes to help remove some of the moisture from the courgettes.

2. Meanwhile, finely grate the zest from the half lemon, then squeeze the juice (keep separate). Stir together all the tzatziki ingredients with the lemon juice and season to taste. Set aside.

3. Transfer the grated courgettes to a clean tea towel, then wrap the towel around it and squeeze out any remaining liquid. In a medium bowl, mix together the flour and egg, then stir through the courgettes, goat's cheese, mint, spring onions, lemon zest and some freshly ground black pepper.

4. Put the oil in a large non-stick frying pan set over a medium heat. Add 3 large spoonfuls of the mixture (spaced well apart) to the pan, spreading each out a little with the back of the spoon. Cook for 3–4 minutes on each side until golden brown and cooked through. Serve with the tzatziki.

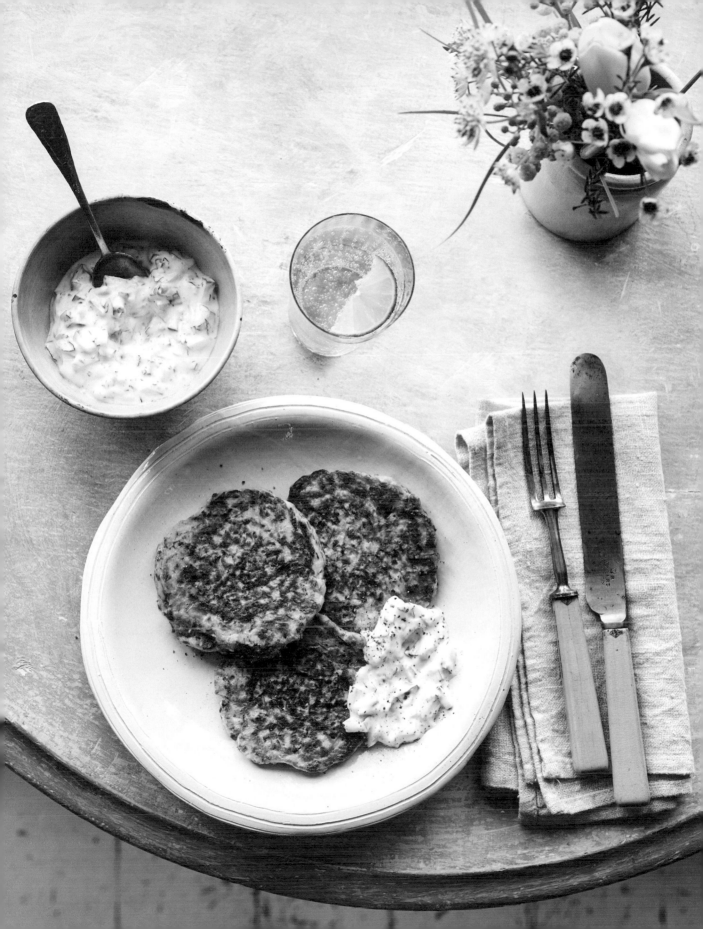

Brown Shrimp and Samphire Tagliatelle

This is the perfect supper to cook for yourself when you're in need of a little indulgence – it's a generous serving of brown shrimp for one, but they make a real treat. If you're doubling up the recipe, the same amount of shrimp will stretch to serve 2.

Hands-on time: 10 minutes
Cooking time: about
** 10 minutes**
Serves 1

75g (3oz) tagliatelle
40g (1½oz) butter
1 shallot, finely chopped
40g (1½oz) samphire, rinsed
  and drained
70g pack brown shrimp
Finely grated zest of 1 lemon,
  plus juice to taste
Pinch of cayenne pepper
100ml (3½fl oz) vegetable
  stock

PER SERVING 650cals,
23g protein, 35g fat (21g
saturates), 57g carbs (4g
total sugars), 7g fibre

1. Cook the pasta in a large pan of boiling water for 10 minutes, or according to the pack instructions, until al dente.

2. Meanwhile, melt the butter in a frying pan over medium heat. Add the shallot and cook for 5 minutes until softened. Turn up the heat to high, then add the samphire, shrimp, lemon zest and cayenne to the pan and fry, stirring, for 2 minutes until the samphire is just tender.

3. Add the stock to the pan and bubble for 2 minutes. Drain the pasta and add to the frying pan. Toss to coat the pasta with the sauce, then season with plenty of freshly ground black pepper and a squeeze of lemon juice. (This dish probably won't need salt as the samphire is naturally salty.) Transfer to a plate or pasta bowl and serve.

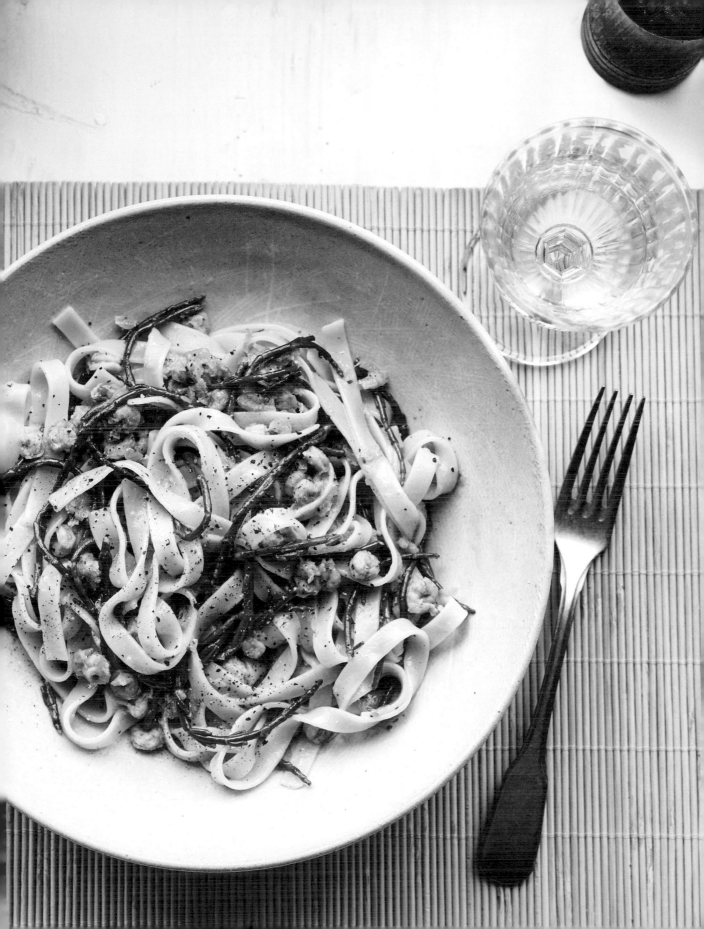

Crusted Cod with Grilled Tomatoes

Use any white fish fillet you like for this low-calorie, simple supper. It goes well with steamed veg and rice or new potatoes for a more substantial meal.

Hands-on time: about 10 minutes
Cooking time: about 10 minutes
Serves 1

1 tsp oil
150g (5oz) boneless cod fillet
1 slice bread
1 tbsp chopped fresh parsley
   or 1 tsp dried mixed herbs
Finely grated zest of ¼ lemon
1 tsp olive oil
75g (3oz) cherry tomatoes on
   the vine

PER SERVING 248cals,
30g protein, 8g fat (1g
saturates), 14g carbs (3g
total sugars), 2g fibre

1. Put the oil in a small frying pan set over a medium heat. Fry the fish, skin-side down, for 3 minutes. Preheat the grill to medium.

2. Meanwhile, coarsely grate the bread or whiz it in a food processor to make crumbs. Put the crumbs into a bowl with the parsley or mixed herbs, lemon zest and olive oil.

3. Carefully lift the part-cooked fish out of the pan and on to a baking sheet. Top with breadcrumb mixture to form a crust. Put the cherry tomatoes on the vine next to the cod, then grill for 5 minutes until the fish is fully cooked and the tomatoes have just burst. Remove from the heat and serve.

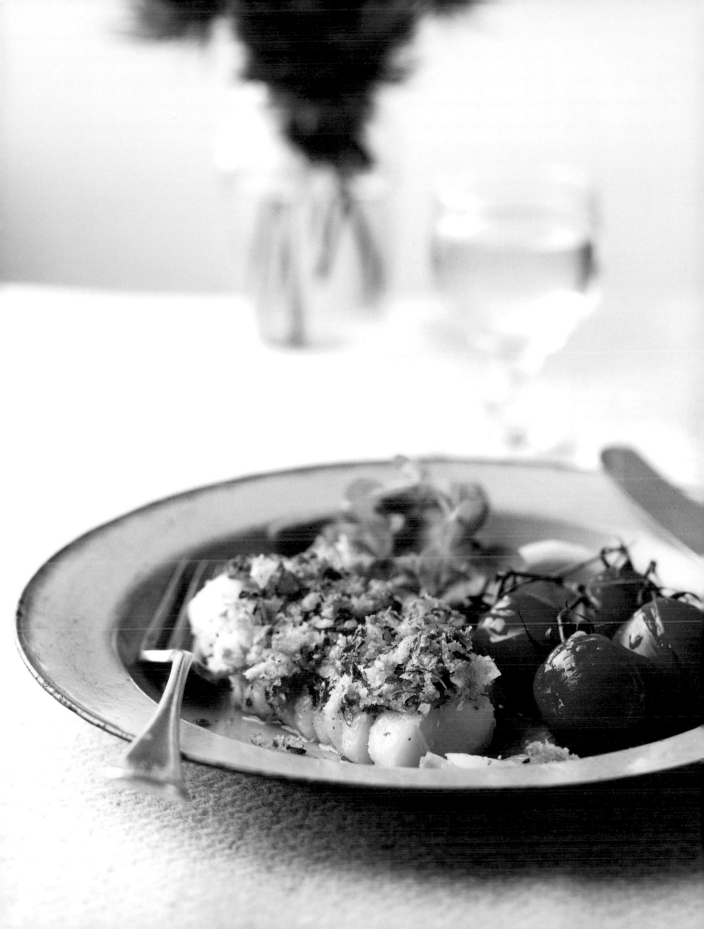

Easy Lamb Tagine

This super-simple version of a Moroccan tagine uses lamb fillets, which cook quickly, to save you time.

Hands-on time: 10 minutes, plus soaking
Cooking time: 20 minutes
Serves 1

1 tsp oil
1 tsp plain flour
150g (5oz) lamb loin fillet, cut into 2.5cm (1in) cubes
½ tsp ground cinnamon
15g (½oz) blanched almonds, roughly chopped
25g (1oz) dried apricots, roughly chopped
200g (7oz) chopped tomatoes
40g (1½oz) couscous
Handful of fresh coriander, chopped, to serve

PER SERVING 614cals, 44g protein, 24g fat (6g saturates), 52g carbs (19g total sugars), 7g fibre

1. Put the oil in a small pan set over a high heat. Sprinkle the flour over the lamb cubes and toss well to coat. Add the lamb cubes to the pan and brown well. Stir in the cinnamon, almonds and apricots, then pour over the chopped tomatoes and enough water to just cover the meat. Simmer gently over a low heat for 15 minutes.

2. Meanwhile, put the couscous into a bowl and pour over just enough boiling water to cover. Cover the bowl with clingfilm and set aside for 10 minutes to soak.

3. When the stew is ready, check the seasoning and fluff up the couscous with a fork. Serve the stew with the couscous, sprinkled with coriander.

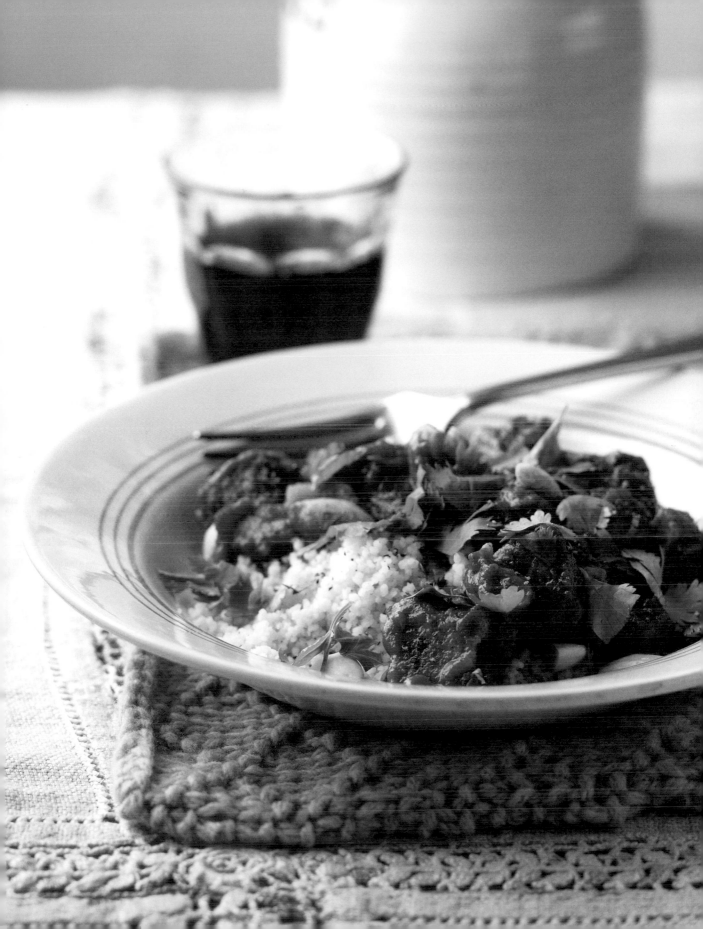

Butterbean Masala

If you're a fan of Indian flavours, garam masala is a storecupboard essential. Conveniently, it's a mixture of spices, so you won't need to keep a collection of spice jars on hand to get an authentic flavour.

Hands-on time: 15 minutes
Cooking time: about
   15 minutes
Serves 1

½ tbsp vegetable oil
1 shallot, sliced
1 garlic clove, crushed
1 tsp garam masala
¼–½ red chilli, deseeded and
  finely chopped
2 tomatoes, roughly chopped
410g tin butterbeans, drained
  and rinsed
Handful of fresh coriander or
  spinach, chopped

PER SERVING 314cals,
16g protein, 8g fat (1g
saturates), 36g carbs (8g
total sugars), 18g fibre

1. Put the vegetable oil in a pan set over medium heat. Gently cook the shallot for 5 minutes. Stir in the garlic, garam masala and chopped chilli, adding more or less depending on how spicy you like your masala, and cook for 1 minute.

2. Add the tomatoes to the pan with 100ml (3½fl oz) water. Simmer for 3 minutes, occasionally squashing the tomatoes with a wooden spoon to help break them down. Stir in the butterbeans and heat through, then stir through the chopped coriander or spinach and check the seasoning. Serve immediately, with rice if you like.

● GH TIPS
This recipe works equally well with chickpeas.

Chilli keeps well in the freezer, so transfer any you don't use to a freezer bag to add to another dish.

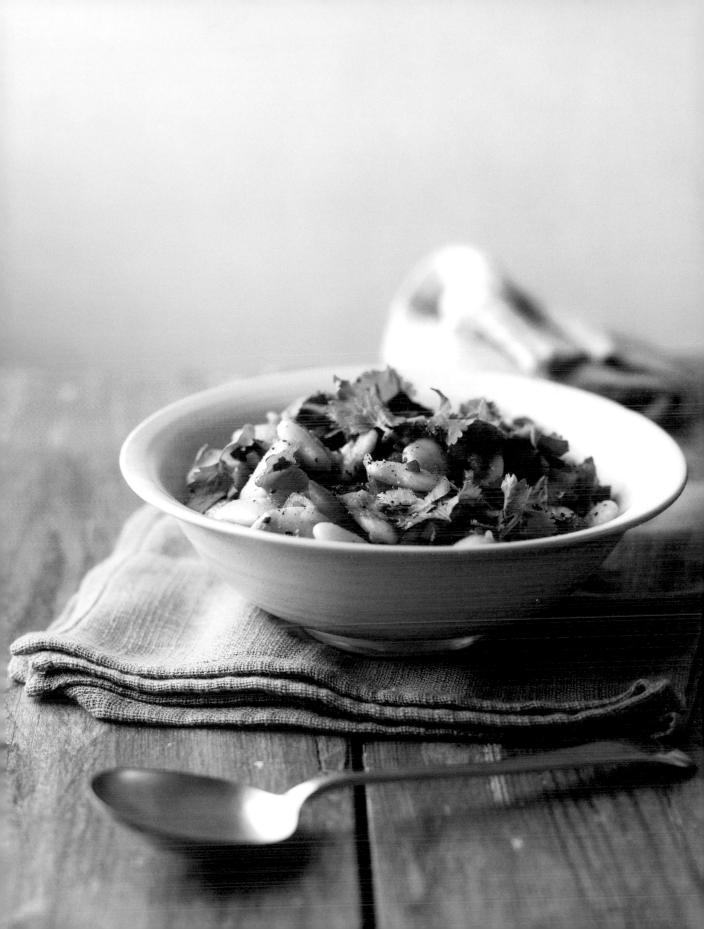

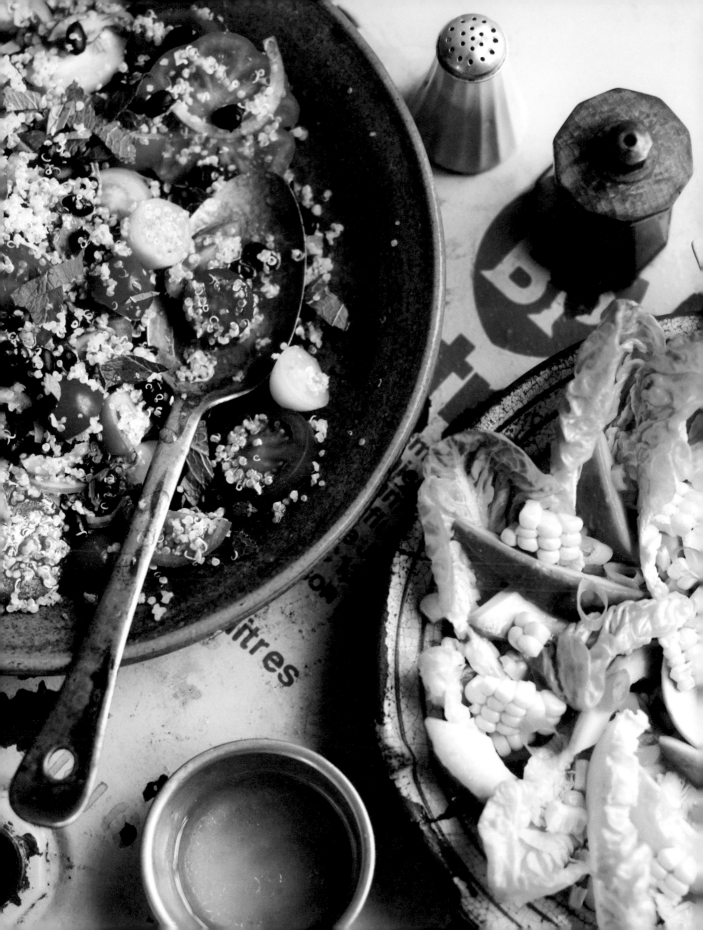

No Cook

Chicken Noodle Soup

Chicken soup normally takes hours to make, but our speedy version is delicious and on the table in minutes.

Hands-on time: 10 minutes
Serves 4

150g (5oz) vermicelli rice
   noodles
2 carrots, cut into fine
   matchsticks
Small bunch of spring onions,
   finely sliced
2 x 195g tins sweetcorn,
   drained
150g (5oz) fresh or frozen peas
4 skinless cooked chicken
   breasts, shredded
2 litres (3½ pints) strong
   gluten-free chicken stock,
   made with boiling water
Small bunch of fresh parsley,
   chopped

PER SERVING 485cals,
53g protein, 3g fat (0g
saturates), 59g carbs (13g
total sugars), 6g fibre

1. In order, put all the ingredients (except the parsley) into a large heatproof bowl or pan. Put a lid on the pan and set it aside for 5 minutes to allow the noodles to soften. Stir in the parsley, season to taste and serve.

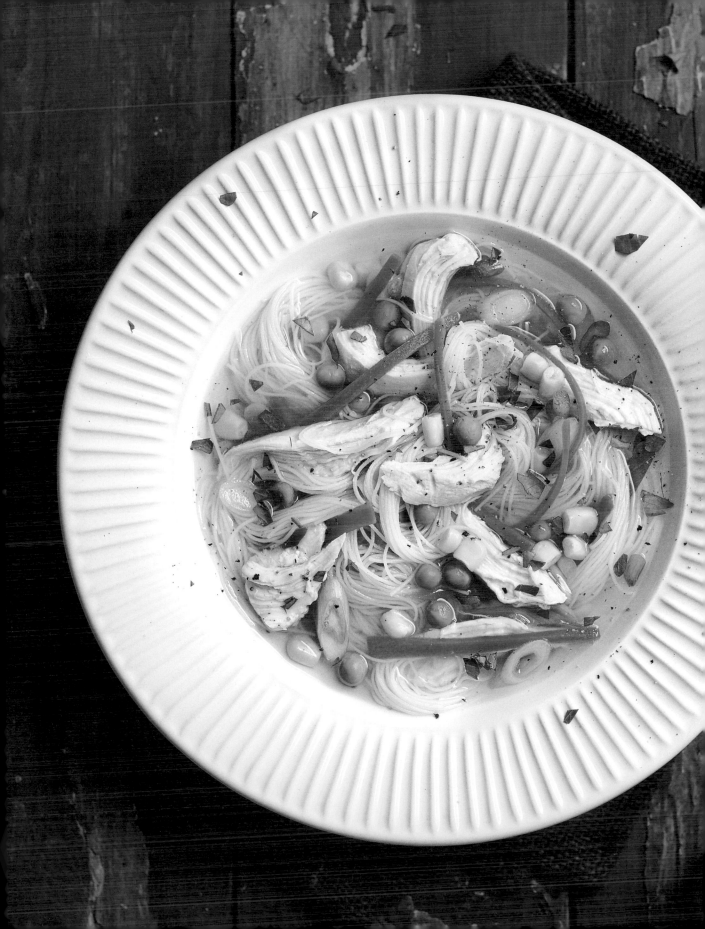

Panzanella

This classic Italian salad makes good use of stale bread and very ripe tomatoes. We've added some butter beans for protein, but feel free to use any tinned pulses you have to hand.

Hands-on time: 15 minutes, plus macerating and soaking
Serves 4

1kg (2lb 3½oz) ripe vine
    tomatoes
½ tsp caster sugar
1 small red onion, finely sliced
2 tbsp sherry vinegar
250g (9oz) stale vegan
    sourdough or ciabatta, torn
    into bite-size pieces
Juice of ½ lemon
100ml (3½fl oz) extra virgin
    olive oil
½ garlic clove, crushed
Large handful of fresh basil,
    leaves picked and torn
15 pitted black olives
2 x 410g tins butterbeans,
    drained and rinsed

PER SERVING 451cals,
12g protein, 22g fat (3g
saturates), 47g carbs (12g
total sugars) 9g fibre

1. Roughly chop the tomatoes, then put into a large serving bowl. Sprinkle over the sugar and a quarter teaspoon salt, then set aside for 15 minutes to allow the juices to be drawn out. In a separate bowl, mix the onion with 1 tablespoon vinegar. Set aside to soften for 15 minutes.

2. When the onion is soft, add the bread to the serving bowl with the tomatoes in it, then tip in the onion mixture (set aside the empty onion bowl). Toss together and leave to soak for 10 minutes.

3. In the reserved empty onion bowl, whisk together the remaining vinegar, lemon juice, oil and some seasoning. Pour half of the mixture into the serving bowl along with the garlic, basil, olives and butterbeans. Stir to combine (if you have time, set aside for a further 15 minutes to allow the flavours to mingle), then serve with the extra dressing alongside.

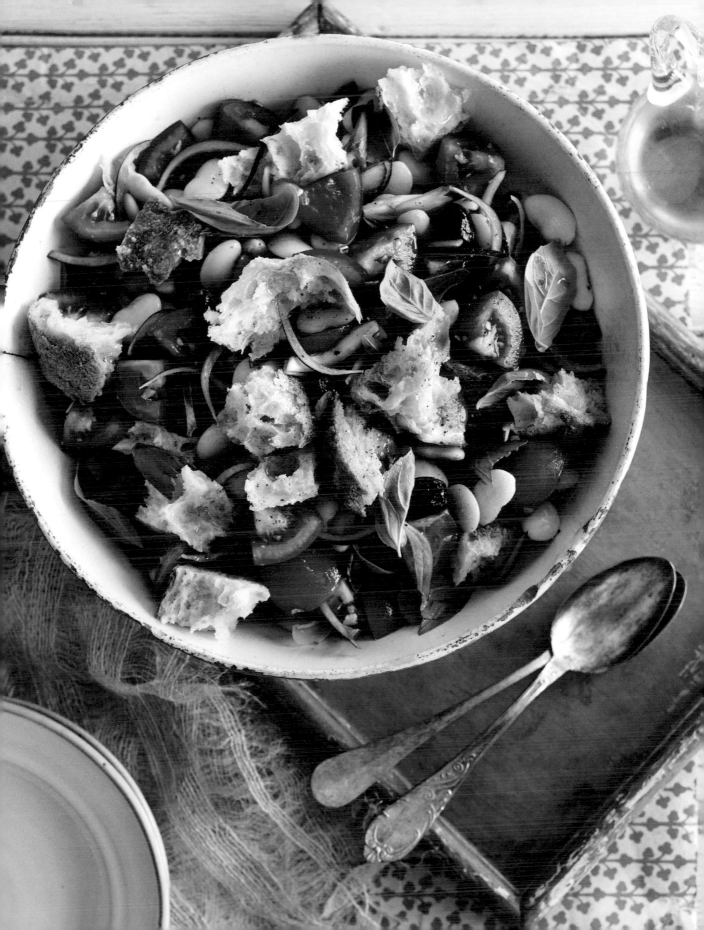

Sweetcorn Chowder with Smoked Mackerel

Blitzing sweetcorn with hot stock, cashews and herbs creates a deliciously creamy soup that's also dairy free.

Hands-on time: 15 minutes
Serves 4

1 gluten-free vegetable
    stock cube
75g (3oz) cashew nuts
2 x 340g tins sweetcorn,
    drained
Small bunch of fresh parsley,
    chopped
Small bunch of fresh chives,
    snipped
225g (8oz) smoked mackerel,
    skinned and flaked

PER SERVING 482cals,
19g protein, 28g fat (6g
saturates), 36g carbs (13g
total sugars), 4g fibre

1. Dissolve the stock cube in 600ml (1 pint) freshly boiled water from the kettle. Set aside a few of the cashew nuts, 1 tablespoon of sweetcorn and some of the herbs to use as a garnish.

2. Pour the stock into a blender, then add the remaining cashews, sweetcorn and herbs. Blend until smooth, then check the seasoning.

3. Divide the soup among 4 warm bowls and top with the mackerel. Serve garnished with the reserved cashews, sweetcorn and herbs.

● GH TIP
Not a fan of smoked mackerel? Add crispy bacon, if you prefer, to the top of this chowder. For a vegetarian option, avocado also works well.

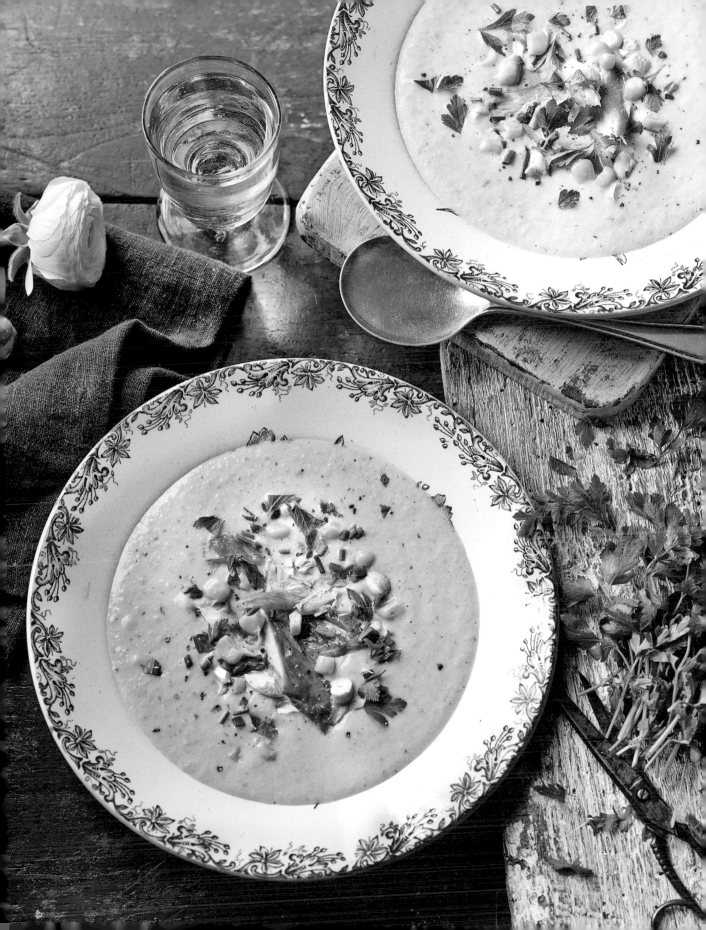

Scandi-style Chopped Salad

Use hot-smoked salmon rather than mackerel, if you prefer, for this fresh and flavoursome recipe.

Hands-on time: 15 minutes, plus pickling
Serves 4

4 tbsp white wine vinegar
1 tsp sugar
Small bunch of fresh dill, chopped
1 cucumber
200g (7oz) radishes, finely sliced
2 celery sticks, sliced
3 spring onions, sliced
75g (3oz) walnuts, roughly chopped
4 tbsp natural yogurt
230g (8oz) smoked mackerel fillets
Gluten-free or rye bread, to serve (optional)

PER SERVING 373cals, 16g protein, 31g fat (5g saturates), 6g carbs (6g total sugars), 2g fibre

1. In a large bowl, mix together the vinegar, sugar, half the dill and a large pinch of salt. Using a mandoline or sharp knife, finely slice the cucumber and add it to the bowl. Mix together gently, then set aside for 15 minutes to pickle lightly.

2. To the cucumber bowl, add the radishes, celery, spring onions, walnuts, yogurt and remaining dill. Peel off and discard any skin from the fish, then flake it into bowl. Fold all the ingredients together and check the seasoning. Serve with gluten-free or rye bread, if you like.

Sweetcorn and Avocado Salad

If you have the time to grill 4 cobs of corn — or have some leftover from a barbecue — adding shards of sweetcorn kernels carved from a cob rather than tinned sweetcorn will make this salad look extra special.

Hands-on time: 10 minutes
Serves 8, as a side salad

2 x 198g tins sweetcorn, drained or 4 sweetcorn cobs, grilled
Juice of 2 limes
3 ripe avocadoes, sliced
A few drops of Tabasco sauce
1 tbsp agave syrup or honey (for non-vegans)
3 Little Gem lettuces, leaves separated
3 spring onions, finely chopped

PER SERVING 225cals, 5g protein, 13g fat (3g saturates), 20g carbs (4g total sugars), 5g fibre

1. Carve off shards of kernels from the sweetcorn cobs. Set aside.

2. Sprinkle half the lime juice over the avocado slices to stop them going brown. Put the remaining lime juice, Tabasco sauce and agave syrup or honey in a small bowl, whisk to combine and season well.

3. Assemble the salad, layering up the ingredients in a wide, shallow bowl. Pour over the dressing and serve.

● GH TIP
Add Tabasco sauce to taste, one drop at a time, as it packs a spicy punch!

Favela Frejola Salad

Microwaveable quinoa pouches are handy cupboard standbys and a wonderful way to give a protein boost to salads.

Hands-on time: 15 minutes
Serves 8, as a side salad

1kg (2lb 3½oz) mixed
    colourful tomatoes, halved
    or sliced if large
2 x 250g pouches ready-
    cooked quinoa
Large bunch of fresh
    tarragon, roughly chopped
Large bunch of fresh mint,
    roughly chopped
1 small red onion, finely
    sliced
2 x 400g tins black beans,
    drained and rinsed

FOR THE DRESSING
2 tsp caster sugar
6 tbsp extra virgin olive oil
Juice of 4 limes

PER SERVING (for 8) 283cals,
11g fat (1g saturates), 32g
carbs (8g total sugars), 9g
protein, 9g fibre

1. Put the tomatoes into a serving bowl. Add the remaining salad ingredients and toss together gently to combine.

2. Whisk all the dressing ingredients together and drizzle over the salad to serve.

◆ GET AHEAD
Make the salad 30 minutes before you eat it and leave it at room temperature to let the flavours develop.

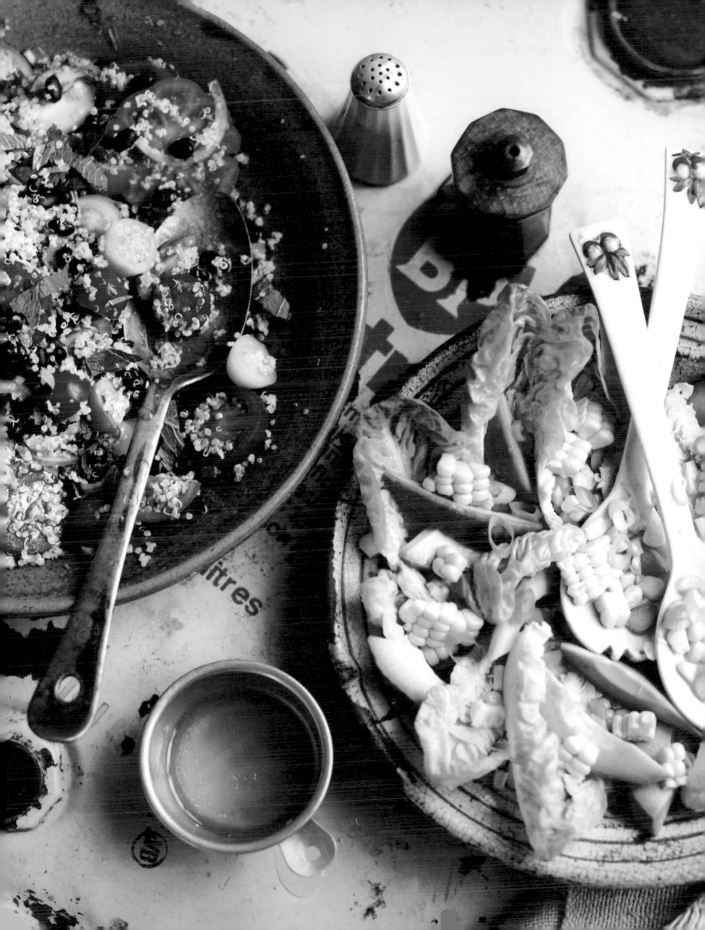

Peach, Ham and Burrata Salad

If you can't get hold of burrata, use two 125g (4oz) balls of torn mozzarella instead. Make this salad throughout the summer months, when fresh peaches are at their best. Other ripe stone-fruit will also work well.

Hands-on time: 10 minutes
Serves 4

3 x 400g tins green lentils, drained and rinsed
4 tbsp extra virgin olive oil, plus extra to drizzle
2 tbsp red wine vinegar
Pinch of sugar
175g (6oz) ham hock or cooked ham, shredded
3 ripe peaches or nectarines, de-stoned and roughly chopped
Small bunch of fresh basil, leaves torn
200g pack burrata, drained

PER SERVING 494cals, 33g protein, 24g fat (9g saturates), 32g carbs (9g total sugars), 9g fibre

1. In a large bowl, mix together all the ingredients except the burrata. Season, then transfer to a serving platter.

2. Lay the burrata over the salad. Break it into quarters just before serving to allow the creamy juices to coat some of the salad.

3. To serve, drizzle with olive oil and sprinkle over some freshly ground black pepper.

● GH TIP
To make a vegetarian version of this salad, omit the ham, check the burrata is vegetarian and add some ready-cooked vegetable antipasti such as artichokes or sun-blush tomatoes

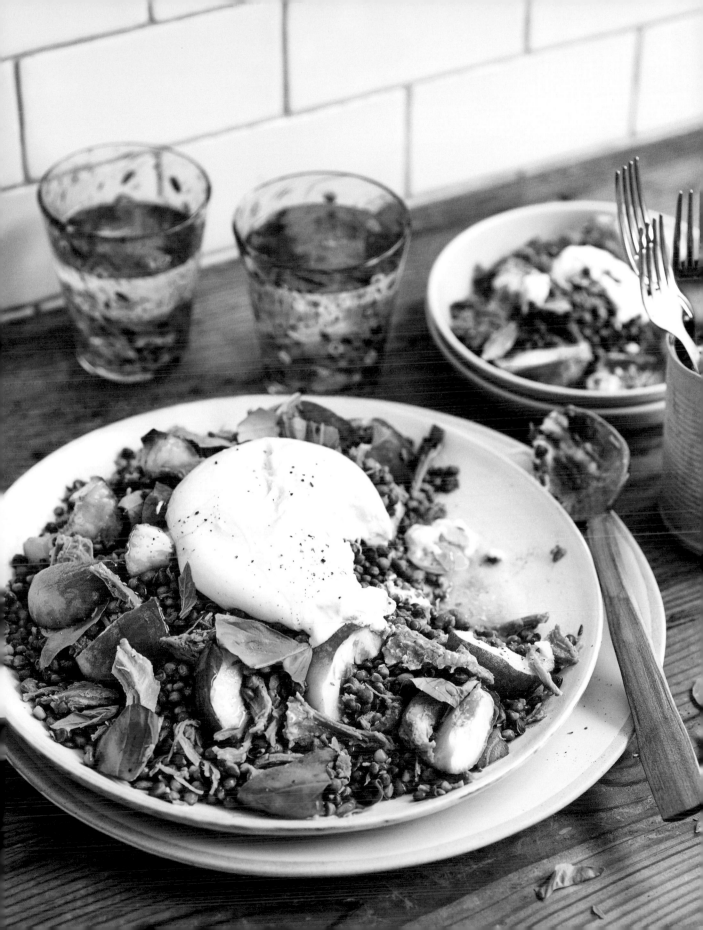

No-cook Bean Burger

This tasty burger is not only vegan, but it requires absolutely no cooking!

Hands-on time: 25 minutes, plus chilling
Serves 8

400g tin kidney beans, drained
400g tin black beans, drained
½ tsp ground cumin
2 tbsp chipotle paste
4 spring onions, trimmed and roughly chopped
Small bunch of coriander, roughly chopped
150g (5oz) roasted red peppers from a jar, drained
75g (3oz) crispy fried onions, crushed
250g pouch ready-cooked quinoa
100g (3½ oz) cherry tomatoes
Pinch of sugar
8 vegan burger buns
2 Little Gem lettuces, leaves separated

PER SERVING 318cals, 13g protein, 9g fat (3g saturates), 44g carbs (4g total sugars), 8g fibre

1. In a food processor, whiz the beans, cumin, chipotle paste, spring onions, half the coriander and 50g (2oz) of the red peppers to make a thick, coarse purée.

2. Tip the purée into a large mixing bowl and stir through the remaining coriander, 25g (1oz) of the crispy fried onions and the cooked quinoa. Season to taste, then form into 8 evenly sized patties. Transfer the burgers to a plate, then cover and chill them for at least 20 minutes to firm up.

3. Roughly chop the remaining red peppers and the cherry tomatoes and put them into a serving bowl with the sugar and some seasoning.

4. Split the buns and toast the halves in a toaster. Meanwhile, scatter the remaining crispy fried onions on a plate. Set the burgers on top and use your fingers to help you press some onion crumbs on to the outside of the burgers. Serve the burgers in the buns with a few lettuce leaves and the red pepper salsa.

◆ GET AHEAD
Prepare the burgers to the end of step 2, then cover and chill for up to 3 days. Complete the recipe to serve.

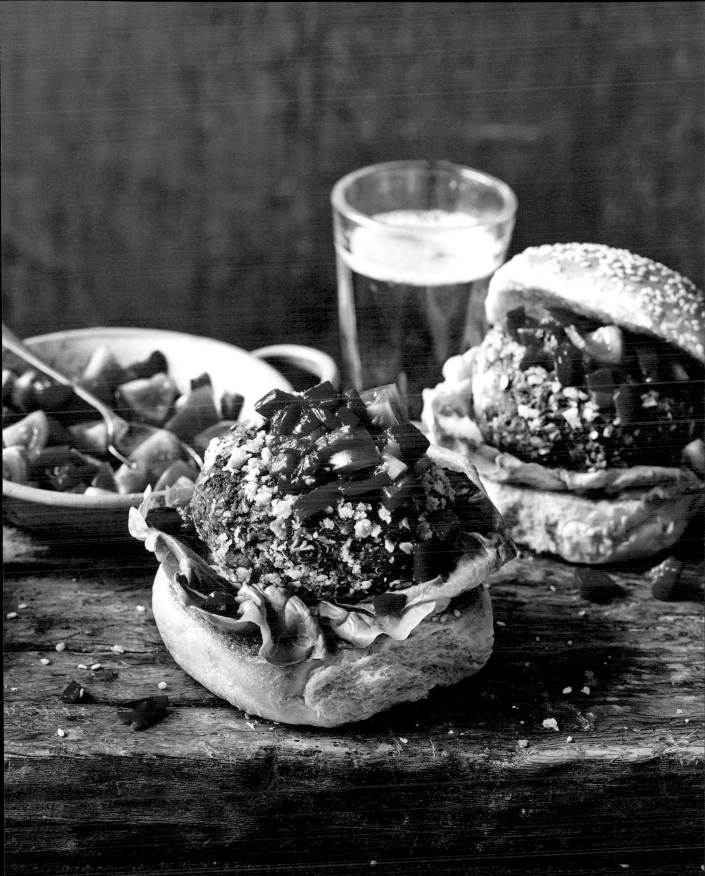

Ceviche

This recipe relies on acid to 'cook' the fish, so make sure you buy super fresh, sustainably sourced fish.

Hands-on time: 10 minutes, plus 'cooking'
Serves 6

500g (1lb 2oz) firm-fleshed, skinned white fish
175ml (6fl oz) lemon juice (about 5 lemons)
1 red onion, finely sliced
200g (7oz) cherry tomatoes, halved
1 green chilli, deseeded and finely chopped
Large handful of fresh coriander, roughly chopped
1 punnet cress, snipped
Extra virgin olive oil, to drizzle

PER SERVING (without extra oil) 88cals, 17g protein, 1g fat (0g saturates), 3g carbs (3g total sugars), 1g fibre

1. Remove any bones in the fish, then cut it into 1cm (½in) cubes. Put the fish into a large non-metallic bowl and add the lemon juice, onion and a quarter teaspoon salt (optional). Leave the fish to 'cook' for 5–30 minutes, depending on whether you prefer fish more raw or 'cooked' through. Stir gently from time to time to make sure the fish remains coated in the liquid.

2. To serve, lift the fish and onions out of the liquid (reserving the liquid) and arrange on a large platter. Dot around the tomatoes, then scatter over the chilli, coriander and cress. Season with freshly ground black pepper. Spoon over a little of the reserved lemon liquid (discard the remainder) and drizzle with extra virgin oil.

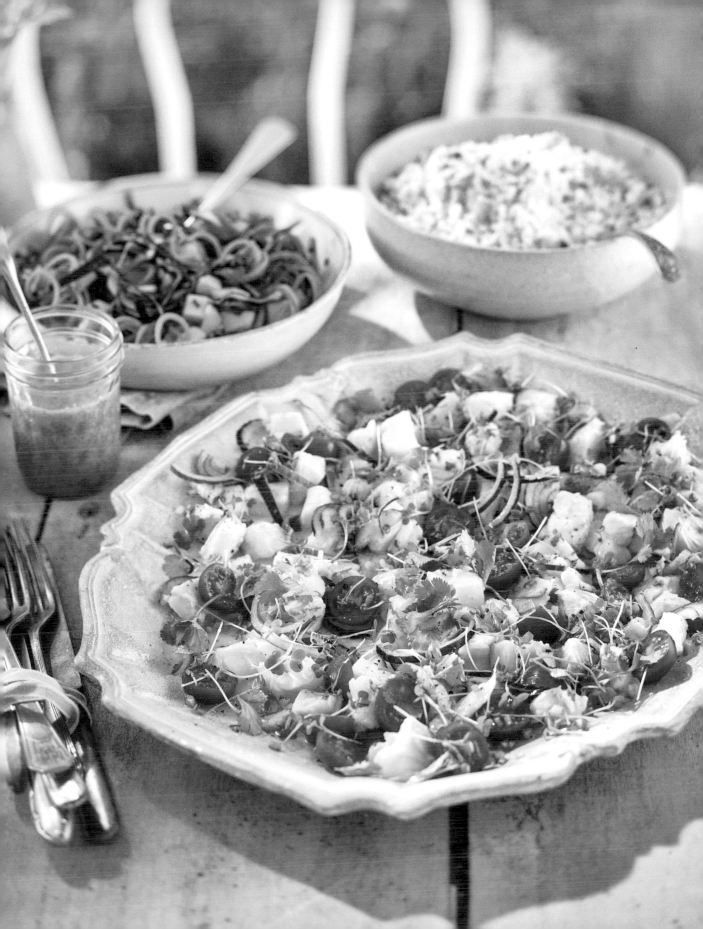

Pistachio-crumbed Goat's Cheese Salad

Look out for different varieties of raw beetroot, such as candy and golden beetroot, to add a colourful touch to this sophisticated salad.

Hands-on time: 10 minutes
Serves 4

2 raw beetroot, trimmed
    and peeled
3 cooked beetroot (from a
    vacuum pack)
Juice of 1 lemon
Pinch of sugar
50g (2oz) pistachio kernels,
    finely chopped
2 x 150g logs soft (rindless)
    goat's cheese
2 carrots, peeled into ribbons
100g (3½oz) lamb's lettuce
3 tbsp extra virgin olive oil
2 tbsp balsamic glaze

PER SERVING 495cals,
22g protein, 35g fat (16g
saturates), 20g carbs (18g
total sugars), 7g fibre

1. With a mandoline or sharp knife, thinly slice the raw and cooked beetroot, keeping them separate. In a medium bowl, mix the raw beetroot with the lemon juice and sugar. Set aside to cure.

2. Scatter half the pistachios over a plate. Roll the outside of the cheese logs in the pistachios to coat them, reserving any excess nuts. Cut each log into 6 even rounds.

3. Remove the raw beetroot from the bowl, reserving the liquid. Divide the raw and cooked beetroot, the carrots and lamb's lettuce among 4 plates. Top each plate with 3 slices of goat's cheese .

4. Add the olive oil and balsamic glaze to the bowl with the beetroot liquid and whisk together. Season and drizzle a little over each salad plate. Sprinkle over the remaining pistachios and serve.

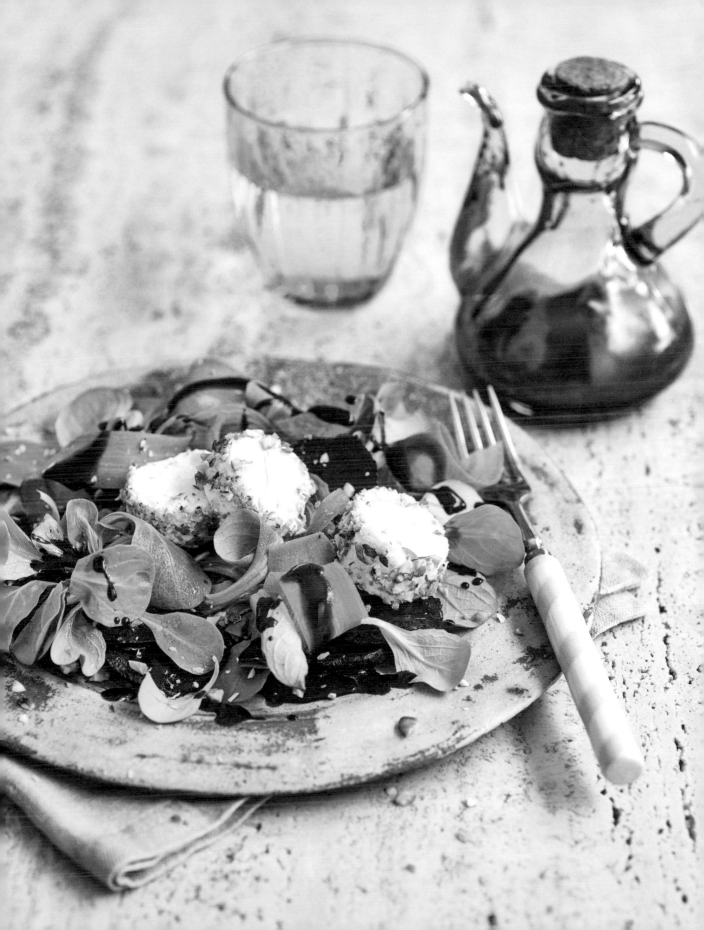

Thai Prawn and Sprouted Bean Salad

Sprouting beans and grains boosts their vitamin content and makes them easier to absorb. They also make a great addition to this super-healthy salad.

Hands-on time: 15 minutes
Serves 4

150g (5oz) vermicelli rice
  noodles
1 large carrot, peeled and
  chopped into matchsticks
100g (3½oz) sugar snap peas,
  roughly chopped
100g (3½oz) mixed sprouted
  beans and grains
2 spring onions, finely sliced
½–1 red chilli, deseeded and
  finely chopped
250g (9oz) cooked king
  prawns
Large handful of fresh
  coriander, roughly chopped
Small handful of fresh mint,
  finely chopped

FOR THE DRESSING
Juice of 2 limes
½ tsp Thai fish sauce
2 tbsp light soy sauce
2 tsp light brown soft sugar

PER SERVING 203cals, 1g fat
(0g saturates), 38g carbs (7g
total sugars), 11g protein,
2g fibre

1. Put the noodles into a bowl and cover with just-boiled water. Set aside to soften for 5 minutes, then drain and rinse under cold water. Return the noodles to the bowl and mix in the carrot, sugar snap peas, sprouted beans and grains, spring onions, chilli and prawns. Stir through the coriander and mint.

2. To make the dressing, whisk together all the ingredients. Pour the dressing over the salad and toss to combine. Serve straight away or chill for up to a day ahead.

● GH TIP
If you can't find sprouted beans and grains, replace them with 100g (3½oz) soya beans.

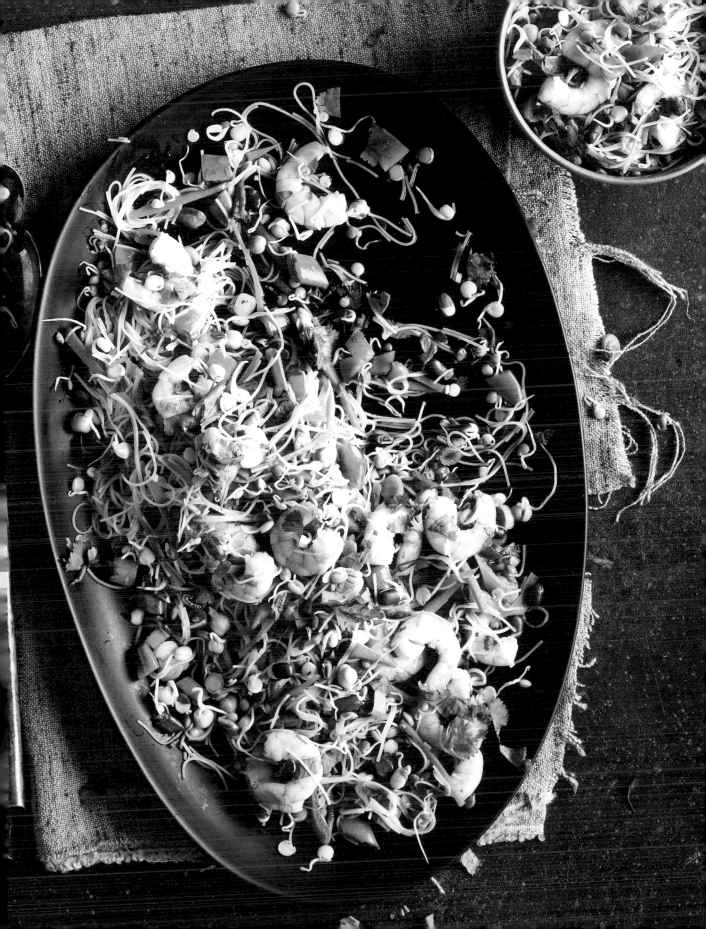

Mexican-style Corn Wraps

Wrapped up in foil, these wraps are great in packed lunches or for a picnic.

Hands-on time: 20 minutes
Serves 4

410g tin kidney beans, drained
    and rinsed
50g (2oz) soured cream
Juice of ½ lemon
½ x 198g tin sweetcorn,
    drained
¼–½ red onion, finely
    chopped, to taste
125g (4oz) cherry tomatoes,
    halved
2 tbsp tomato ketchup
½–1 tsp chipotle paste
Large handful of fresh
    coriander leaves, roughly
    chopped
4 large flour tortilla wraps
¼ iceberg lettuce, shredded
75g (3oz) mature vegetarian
    Cheddar cheese, grated

PER SERVING 408cals,
11g fat (6g saturates), 64g
carbs (10g total sugars), 17g
protein, 8g fibre

1. Whiz the beans, soured cream, lemon juice and plenty of seasoning in a food processor until smooth. Set aside.

2. Put the sweetcorn kernels into a large bowl. Add the red onion, cherry tomatoes, ketchup, chipotle paste and coriander. Stir to combine and check the seasoning.

3. Put a wrap on a board and smear a quarter of the bean purée in a line along the centre, leaving a 5cm (2in) border at each end. Top with a quarter each of the lettuce, sweetcorn mixture and Cheddar. Fold the sides of the wrap over the filling, then roll up to enclose, securing the wrap in place with a cocktail stick, if you like. Slice the wraps in half and serve.

● GH TIP
To make this meaty, pan-fry sliced chicken breast with some fajita seasoning and add to the wrap before rolling up.

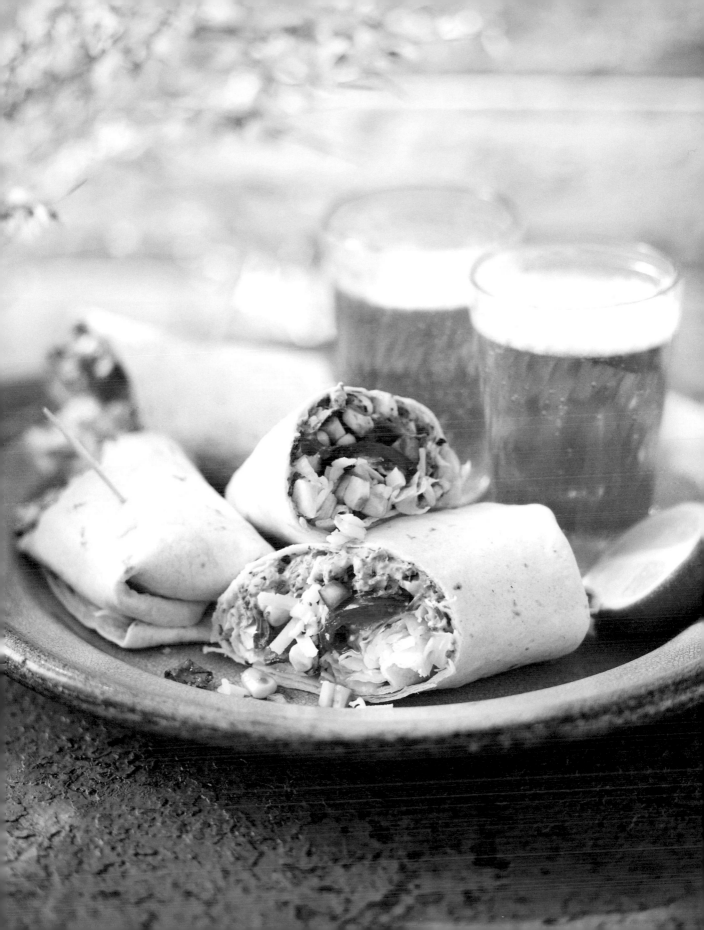

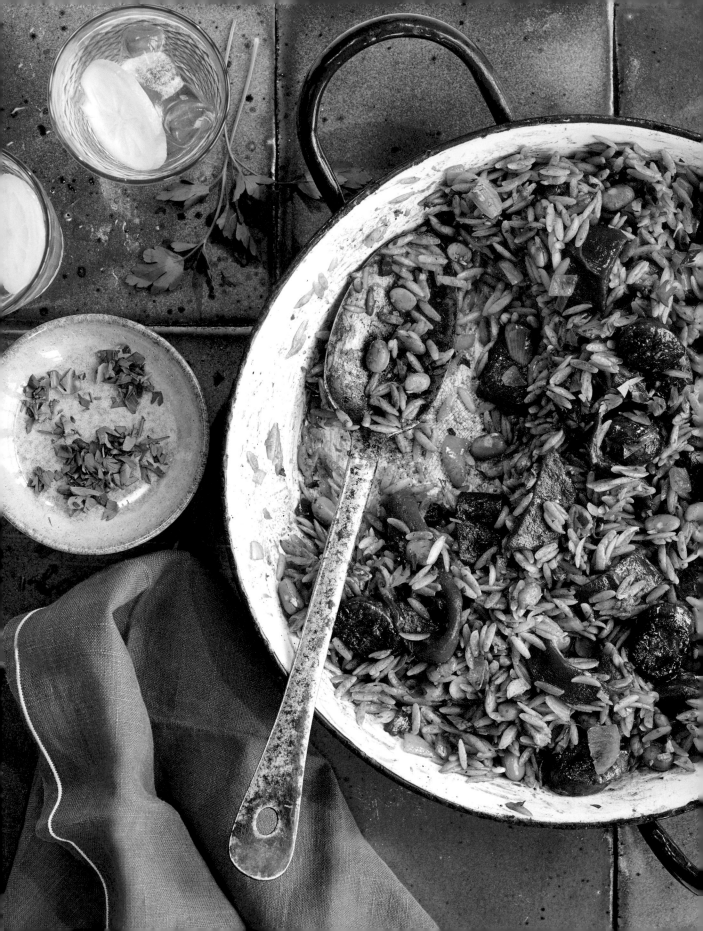

5

One Pot

Speedy Chicken Laksa

You can use a green Thai curry paste rather than red, if you prefer.

Hands-on time: 5 minutes
Cooking time: 10 minutes
Serves 4

1–2 tbsp red Thai curry paste,
    to taste
1 litre (1¾ pints) chicken stock
400ml tin coconut milk
3 cooked skinless chicken
    breasts
150g (5oz) medium egg
    noodles
150g (5oz) beansprouts
5 spring onions, sliced
1 red chilli, finely sliced
Handful of fresh coriander,
    roughly chopped

PER SERVING 557cals,
45g protein, 25g fat (17g
saturates), 37g carbs (5g
total sugars), 3g fibre

1. Set a large, deep frying pan over medium heat and fry the curry paste for 30 seconds until fragrant. Add the stock and coconut milk and bring to the boil.

2. Meanwhile, use your fingers to shred the chicken into bite-size strips.

3. Add the noodles to the pan and bubble for 4 minutes until tender, then stir in the shredded chicken, beansprouts and most of the spring onions. Heat through and check the seasoning.

4. Divide among 4 bowls and garnish with the remaining spring onions, sliced chilli and coriander.

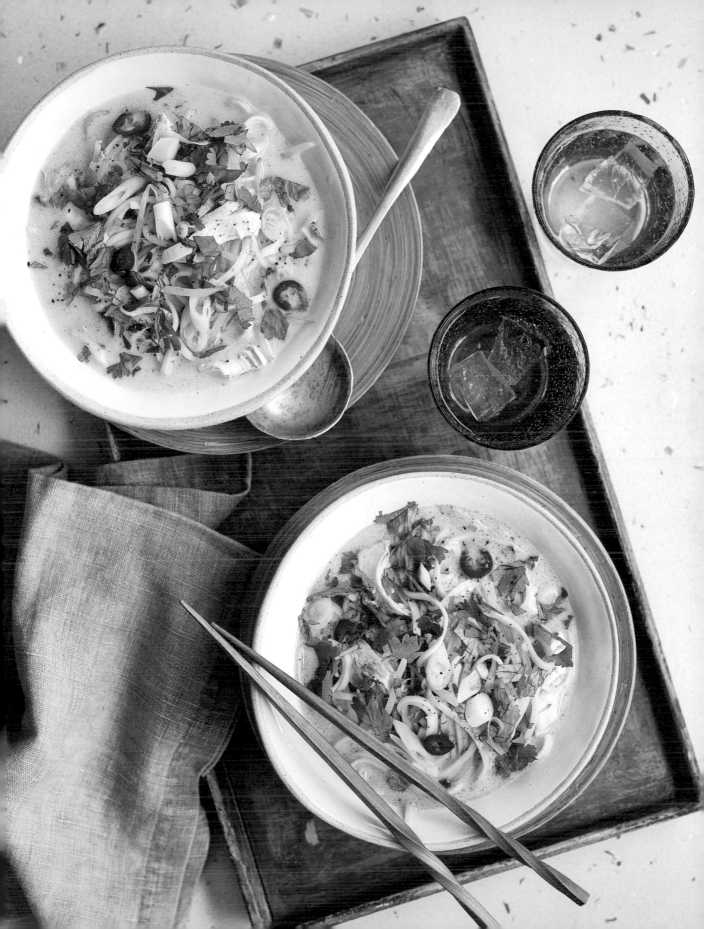

Green Shakshuka

This one-pan supper takes its cue from the Middle-Eastern dish of eggs cooked in a spicy tomato and chilli sauce. This version features spring greens and fresh, herby flavours for a seasonal twist.

Hands-on time: 15 minutes
Cooking time: about
   20 minutes
Serves 4

1 tbsp olive oil
300g (11oz) leftover cooked
   new potatoes, sliced
300g (11oz) mixed spring
   greens, spinach and chard
1 garlic clove, chopped
2 tsp cumin seeds
A small handful each of fresh
   mint, parsley and dill,
   chopped
200g (7oz) frozen peas,
   defrosted
4 eggs
Natural yogurt and flatbreads,
   to serve

PER SERVING 216cals,
13g protein, 9g fat (2g
saturates), 18g carbs (5g
total sugars), 7g fibre

1. Put the oil in a large frying pan set over medium heat. Fry the new potatoes for 5 minutes until turning golden, then add the greens and cook for a further 3–4 minutes until wilted. Stir in the garlic, cumin, most of the fresh herbs, peas and plenty of seasoning, then cover and cook for a few minutes more.

2. Make 4 wells in the mixture and crack an egg into each. Cover the pan and cook for 5–6 minutes until the egg whites are just set, then season with black pepper. Remove from the heat, sprinkle with the remaining herbs and serve with a dollop of natural yogurt and flatbreads, if you like.

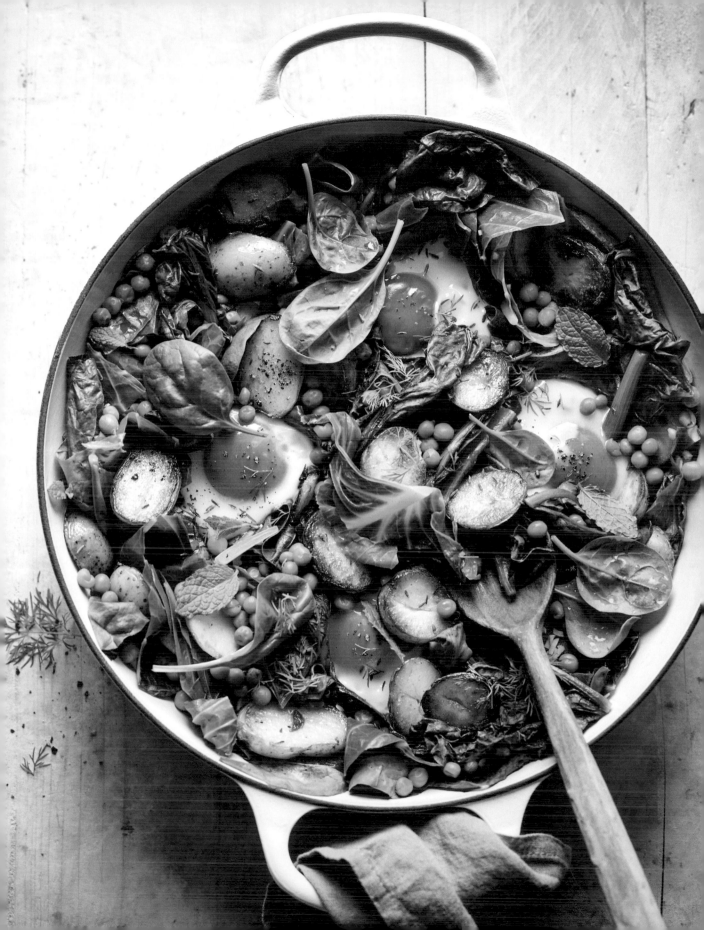

Hot-and-sour Pork Broth

A clean and sprightly broth that is ideal for a light supper. Replace the pork with the same weight of skinless chicken breast, if you prefer.

Hands-on time: 10 minutes
Cooking time: 15 minutes
Serves 4

200g (7oz) flat rice noodles
1 tbsp groundnut or vegetable oil
125g (4oz) shiitake mushrooms, sliced
2 garlic cloves, finely sliced
5cm (2in) piece fresh root ginger, cut into matchsticks
2 litres (3½ pints) chicken stock
350g (12oz) pork fillet, cut into strips
150g (5oz) sugar snap peas, sliced lengthways
2 tbsp rice vinegar
2 tbsp soy sauce
1–2 tsp sriracha hot chilli sauce, to taste
Spring onions, finely sliced, to garnish
Fresh coriander, chopped, to garnish
Red chilli, finely sliced, to garnish (optional)

PER SERVING 511cals, 44g protein, 9g fat (2g saturates), 62g carbs (4g total sugars), 1g fibre

1. Put the noodles in a heatproof bowl and cover with hot water. Soak for about 5–10 minutes until the noodles are pliable.

2. Meanwhile, put the oil in a large pan set over high heat and fry the mushrooms for 2–3 minutes until lightly golden. Add the garlic and ginger and cook for 30 seconds to release their fragrance. Add the stock and bring to the boil.

3. Meanwhile, drain the noodles, then add them to the pan with the pork and sugar snap peas. Bring the broth back to the boil and simmer for 4 minutes until the pork is cooked through. Add the vinegar, soy sauce and sriracha sauce, and check the seasoning.

4. Ladle the broth into bowls to serve and garnish with spring onions, coriander and chilli, if you like.

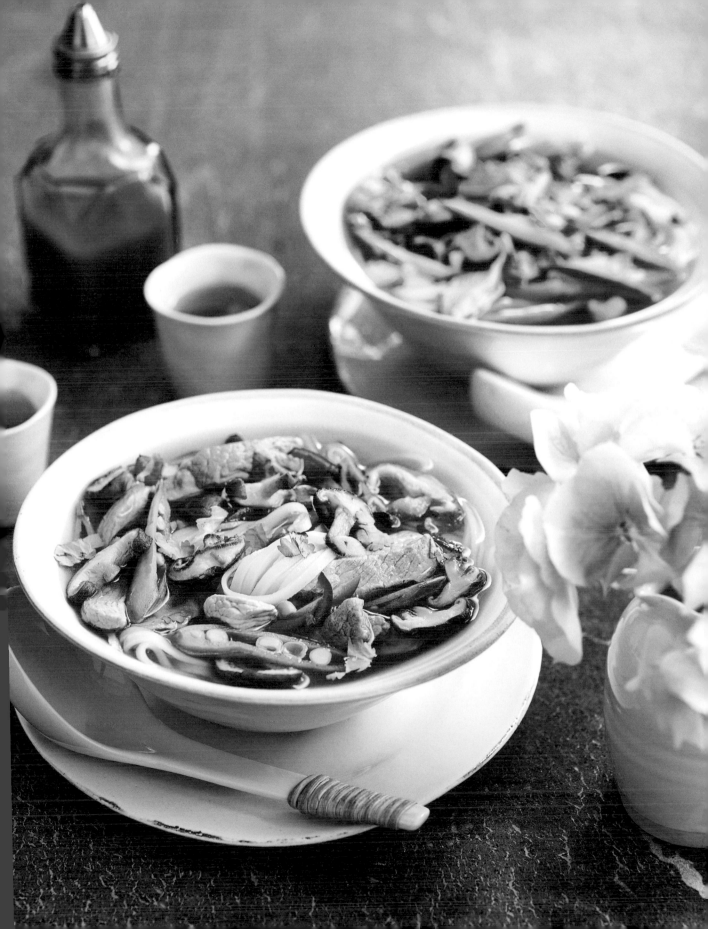

One-pan Fish with Spring Vegetables

This all-in-one meal is easy to assemble, cooks in minutes and has a tangy citrus kick.

Hands-on time: 5 minutes
Cooking time: 12 minutes
Serves 4

125g (4oz) Tenderstem
   broccoli, halved lengthways
250g (9oz) fine asparagus
4 x 125g (4oz) skinless and
   boneless white fish fillets,
   such as haddock, pollock,
   cod or coley
50ml (2fl oz) white wine
1 orange, cut into 8 wedges
75g (3oz) sourdough bread,
   torn into pieces
2 tbsp olive oil
Green salad or boiled rice, to
   serve (optional)

**PER SERVING 227cals,
27g protein, 7g fat (1g
saturates), 11g carbs (2g
total sugars), 3g fibre**

1. Preheat the oven to 220°C (200°C fan) mark 7. Spread the broccoli and asparagus in an even layer over the base of a medium roasting tin. Lay the fish fillets on top and pour over the wine, then tuck in the orange wedges and bread around the fish. Drizzle over the olive oil and season well.

2. Cook in the oven for 10–12 minutes, until the fish is cooked through and the vegetables are just tender (they should still have bite). Serve immediately with some boiled rice or a green salad, if you like.

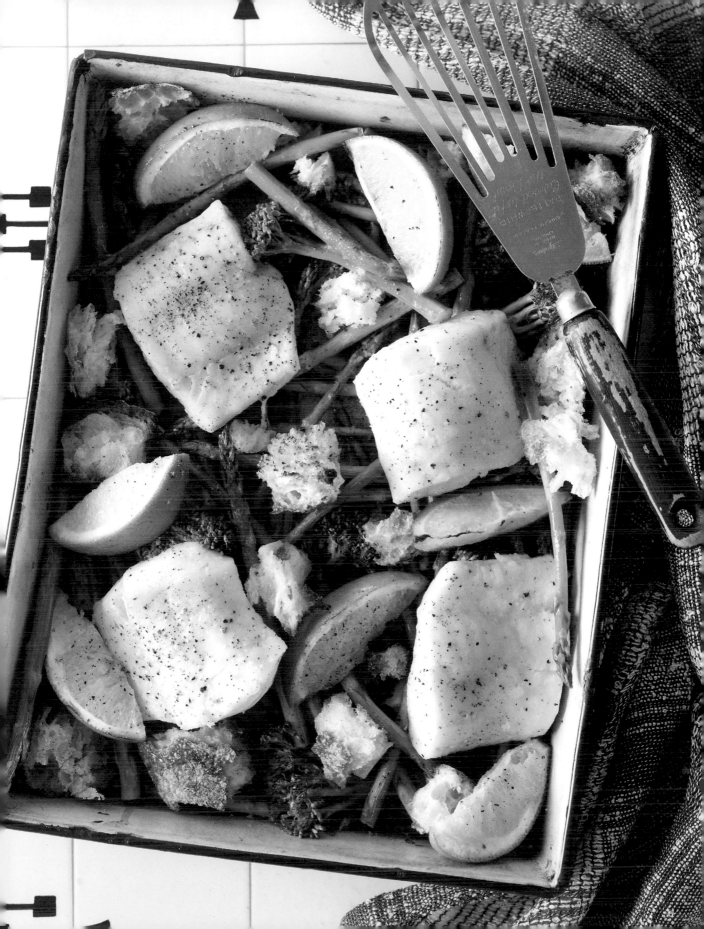

Prawn Gumbo Stew

Go easy on the spice mix if you fancy a milder version of this Cajun classic.

Hands-on time: 10 minutes
Cooking time: about
   15 minutes
Serves 4

1 tbsp oil
Small bunch of spring onions, chopped
2 celery sticks, chopped
2 green peppers, deseeded and cut into 2.5cm (1in) pieces
1 garlic clove, crushed
1½ tbsp Cajun spice mix
1 tbsp plain flour
400ml (14fl oz) chicken stock
400g tin chopped tomatoes
175g (6oz) okra, trimmed and cut into 3cm (1¼in) pieces
300g (11oz) raw king prawns
2 x 250g pouches ready-cooked rice

PER SERVING 371cals, 24g protein, 6g fat (1g saturates), 52g carbs (7g total sugars), 7g fibre

1. Put the oil in a large, deep frying pan (that has a lid) set over medium heat. Fry the white parts of the spring onions (reserve the chopped green tops) with the celery, covering the pan with the lid, for 3 minutes. Add the green peppers and continue to cook, covered, for 4 minutes. Stir in the garlic and Cajun spice mix and heat for 30 seconds, then add the flour and cook for a further 30 seconds.

2. Gradually add the stock, scraping up the bits from the bottom of the pan and stirring until smooth. Stir in the tomatoes. When the mixture is bubbling, add the okra and simmer for 5 minutes, uncovered. Add the prawns and simmer, covered, for 1 minute until the prawns turn pink.

3. Meanwhile, heat the rice according to the pack instructions. Check the seasoning of the gumbo and scatter over the reserved spring onion greens. Serve the gumbo with the rice.

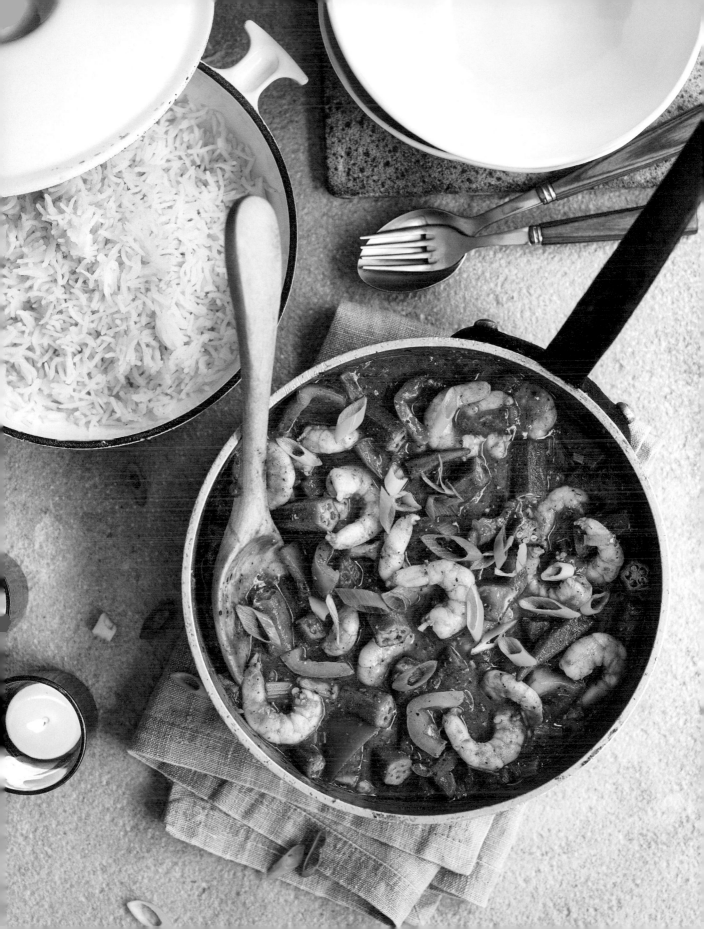

Scandi-style Salmon and New Potato Traybake

Lightly smoked salmon fillets add an extra layer of flavour to this Scandinavian inspired supper, but normal salmon fillets will work equally well. You can also swap the tarragon for dill, if you prefer.

Hands-on time: 10 minutes
Cooking time: about
  25 minutes
Serves 4

2 tbsp rapeseed or sunflower
  oil
750g (1lb 10½oz) baby new
  potatoes
3 tbsp chopped fresh tarragon
  leaves
Juice and zest of 1 lemon,
  plus extra lemon wedges to
  serve
175g (6oz) baby leeks,
  trimmed
2 tsp gluten-free Dijon
  mustard
6 tbsp crème fraîche
1 tbsp capers, drained and
  rinsed
4 x lightly smoked salmon
  fillets
200g (7oz) frozen peas

PER SERVING 608cals,
46g protein, 29g fat (10g
saturates), 38g carbs (9g
total sugars), 7g fibre

1. Preheat the oven to 220°C (200°C fan) mark 7. Pour the oil into a large roasting tin and put in the oven to preheat. Cut the potatoes into evenly sized quarters and carefully transfer to the heated roasting tin. Add 1 tablespoon of the tarragon, half of the lemon zest and some seasoning, then toss the potatoes to coat them in the hot oil. Roast in the oven for 15 minutes.

2. Meanwhile, put the leeks in a bowl and cover with freshly boiled water, set aside for 10 minutes to soak, then drain. For the dressing, whisk together the mustard, crème fraîche (use half-fat crème fraîche, if you prefer), capers, 2 tablespoons lemon juice, 1 tablespoon chopped tarragon and 1 tablespoon water to loosen. Season to taste.

3. After 15 minutes, remove the potatoes from the oven (they should be almost tender – if not, return them to the oven for an extra 5 minutes). Drain the leeks and add these to the potato tin, toss briefly, then top with the salmon. Sprinkle over the remaining tarragon and lemon zest and season well. Scatter over the frozen peas and return the roasting tin to the oven for a further 8–10 minutes until the salmon is cooked through.

4. Remove the tin from the oven and transfer the vegetables and salmon to serving plates. Drizzle with the dressing and serve with lemon wedges to squeeze over.

Spiced-up Salmon Noodles

Better than a take-away, these salmon noodles also make a great packed lunch.

Hands-on time: 10 minutes
Cooking time: about
   10 minutes
Serves 4

1 tbsp vegetable oil
1 large garlic clove, crushed
2.5cm (1in) piece fresh root
  ginger, grated
4 x 150g (5oz) skinless and
  boneless salmon fillets,
  chopped into large pieces
150g (5oz) mangetout
Large pinch of dried chilli
  flakes
75g (3oz) tomato ketchup
2 tbsp soy sauce
2 x 300g packs straight-to-wok
  cooked egg noodles
1 tbsp toasted sesame oil
Large handful of beansprouts
4 spring onions, sliced
Large handful of fresh
  coriander, chopped

PER SERVING 603cals,
42g protein, 27g fat (4g
saturates), 48g carbs (8g
total sugars), 3g fibre

1. Put the vegetable oil in a large frying pan or wok set over a high heat. Fry the garlic and root ginger for 10 seconds until fragrant, then add the salmon pieces and cook for 2–3 minutes until the fish turns opaque.

2. Add the mangetout, chilli flakes, tomato ketchup, soy sauce, noodles and a splash of water to the pan and cook for 4–5 minutes. Gently stir through the sesame oil, beansprouts and most of the spring onions and coriander. Check the seasoning.

3. Divide the noodles among 4 bowls, then garnish with the remaining spring onions and coriander and serve immediately.

Prawn Green Curry Noodles

Packed with flavour, this quick-to-make Thai green curry sauce is a colourful accompaniment to juicy prawns and green veg.

Hands-on time: 5 minutes
Cooking time: 10 minutes
Serves 4

75g (3oz) fresh coriander (leaves and stems), plus extra leaves to garnish
1 garlic clove
3cm (1¼in) piece fresh root ginger
1 green chilli, deseeded and roughly chopped
1 tbsp Thai fish sauce
400ml tin coconut milk
200g (7oz) sugar snap peas
4 x 150g packs straight-to-wok rice noodles
300g (11oz) cooked and peeled king prawns
Juice of 1 lime, plus extra wedges, to serve
Large handful of baby spinach leaves

PER SERVING 543cals, 27g protein, 21g fat (0.2g saturates), 58g carbs (4g total sugars), 6g fibre

1. Put the coriander, garlic, ginger, chilli, fish sauce and coconut milk into a food processor or blender and whiz until smooth.

2. Set a large wok or frying pan over medium heat. Add the coriander mixture and sugar snap peas, then bring to the boil and bubble for 3–5 minutes until the mixture thickens slightly and the sugar snap peas are tender.

3. Add the noodles and prawns and heat through, stirring carefully to separate the noodles without breaking them up. Add the lime juice and season to taste, then fold through the spinach.

4. Divide among 4 bowls, sprinkle with coriander leaves and serve with lime wedges to squeeze over.

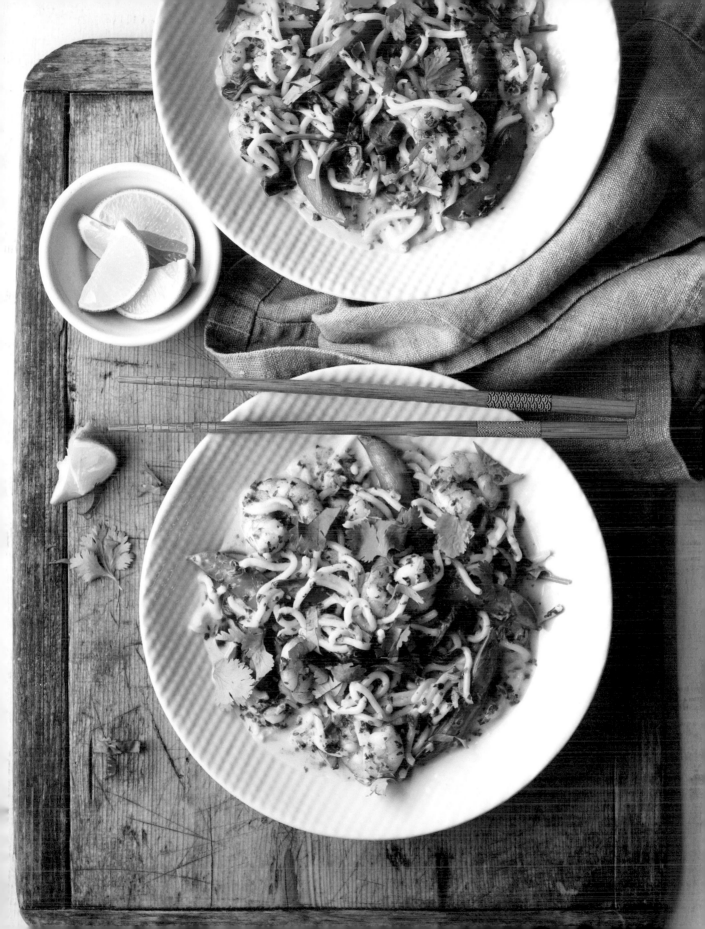

All-in-one Butternut, Bacon and Sage Pasta

One-pan pasta makes a fast, filling and warming midweek meal. Once you've tried it, you'll be hooked!

Hands-on time: 10 minutes
Cooking time: about
  15–20 minutes
Serves 4

300g (11oz) penne pasta

300g (11oz) peeled butternut squash, cut into 1.5cm (⅝in) pieces

2 shallots, finely sliced

4 rashers smoked streaky bacon, sliced

5 whole sage leaves, plus extra leaves, shredded, to garnish

50ml (2fl oz) olive oil

1 litre (1¾ pints) hot chicken stock

40g (1½oz) Parmesan, plus extra to garnish

75ml (3fl oz) double cream

PER SERVING 625cals, 27g protein, 30g fat (12g saturates), 60g carbs (7g total sugars), 5g fibre

1. Into a large, heavy-based pan, put the pasta, squash cubes, shallots, bacon slices, whole sage leaves and oil with some seasoning.

2. Pour over the hot stock and bring to the boil, then turn down the heat slightly and bubble, stirring occasionally, until most of the water has been absorbed and the pasta is just tender. Add the grated cheese and double cream, bubble for a further minute, and check the seasoning.

3. Remove the pasta from the heat and divide it among 4 pasta bowls. Serve sprinkled with some extra grated cheese and shredded fresh sage leaves.

● GH TIP

To make the pasta vegetarian-friendly, leave out the bacon and use a vegetarian hard cheese and stock.

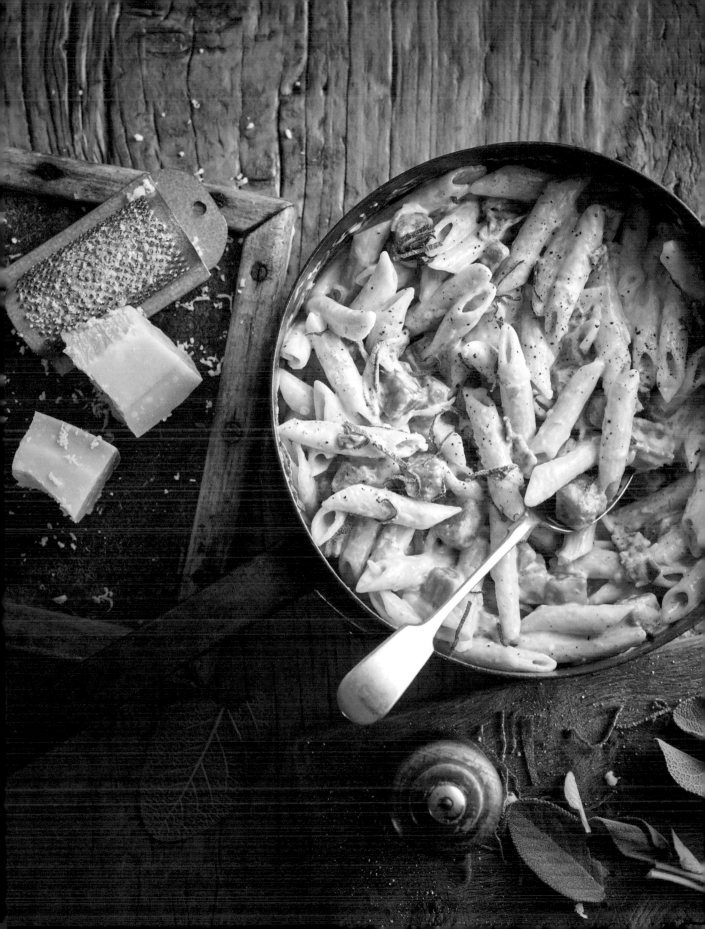

Quick Pork Meatball Cassoulet

This tasty, Italian-inspired meatball and bean stew is an excellent choice for cold winter days.

Hands-on time: 5 minutes
Cooking time: about
  30 minutes
Serves 4

25g (1oz) dried porcini
  mushrooms
1 tbsp olive oil
300g (11oz) ready-made
  pork meatballs
400g pack soffritto mix (or a
  mixture of chopped onion,
  carrot and celery)
2 garlic cloves, finely chopped
4 fresh thyme sprigs, leaves
  removed, plus extra to
  garnish
2 x 400g tins chopped
  tomatoes
400g tin butterbeans, drained
  and rinsed
115g pack baby spinach
Crusty bread, to serve
  (optional)

PER SERVING 341cals,
9g protein, 13g fat (2g
saturates), 44g carbs (3g
total sugars), 4g fibre

1. Put the dried mushrooms into a small bowl, cover with 150ml (5fl oz) boiling water and set aside to soak.

2. Meanwhile, put the oil in a large, deep frying pan set over medium-high heat. Add the meatballs and cook for 5–8 minutes, turning occasionally, until browned all over. Remove to a plate with a slotted spoon and set aside.

3. Keeping the pan over a low to medium heat, add the soffritto mix to the pan and fry for 5 minutes until softened. Add the garlic and thyme leaves and cook for a further 2 minutes to release their aroma. Stir in the porcini mushrooms with the soaking liquid, the chopped tomatoes and some seasoning. Bring to the boil, then turn down to a simmer. Return the meatballs to the pan and continue cooking for around 5 minutes or until the mixture has thickened slightly.

4. Stir in the beans and spinach, and cook the stew for a further 5 minutes to thicken a little more. Sprinkle over some extra fresh thyme and serve with crusty bread, if you like.

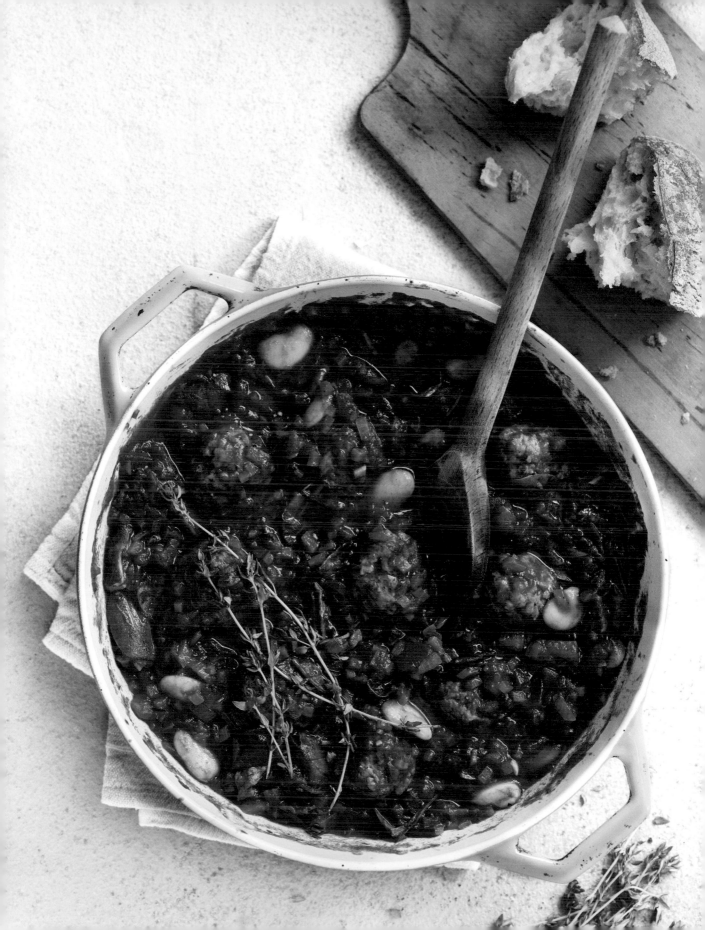

One-pan Lasagne

Using the hob for most of the cooking and adding a great shortcut for white sauce helps you get this favourite on the table in record time.

Hands-on time: 15 minutes
Cooking time: 25 minutes
Serves 6

1 tbsp olive oil
1 onion, finely sliced
500g (1lb 2oz) lean beef mince
500g jar tomato and basil
    pasta sauce
Large bunch of fresh basil,
    roughly chopped
500g (1lb 2oz) ricotta
50g (2oz) Parmesan, grated
1 medium egg, beaten
5–6 large fresh lasagne sheets
75g (3oz) grated mozzarella

**PER SERVING 452cals,
36g protein, 27g fat (13g
saturates), 17g carbs (8g
total sugars) 1g fibre**

1. In a deep, ovenproof frying pan (about 23cm/9in across the base), heat the oil and fry the onion and mince for 5 minutes until the mince is brown and the onion is soft. Stir in the pasta sauce and half the fresh basil, then simmer for 1 minute. Meanwhile, in a medium bowl mix together the ricotta, Parmesan and egg and some seasoning.

2. Scoop two-thirds of the mince mixture out of the pan into a separate bowl. Lay a single layer of lasagne sheets over the mince mixture in the pan (tearing the sheets, if needed, to fit). Spoon over one-third of the ricotta mixture and a sprinkling of mozzarella. Repeat these layers twice more (adding mince from bowl), finishing with a layer of ricotta on top and a sprinkling of grated mozzarella. Cover the pan with a lid or baking sheet, and simmer on the hob for 10–12 minutes.

3. Heat the grill to high. Once the pasta is tender, put the pan under the grill for 3–5 minutes until golden. Sprinkle over the remaining basil and some freshly ground pepper, then serve.

● GH TIP
Prefer moussaka? Swap the beef for lamb mince, adding 1 teaspoon ground cinnamon to the mixture, and use feta instead of mozzarella.

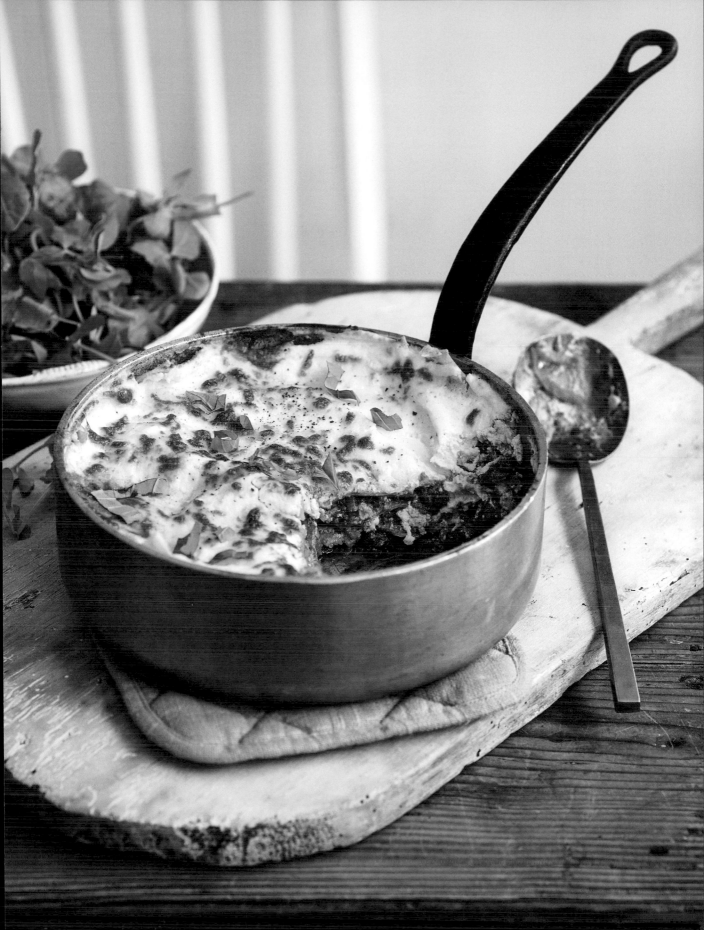

Turkey Pad Thai

This traditional Thai street food dish is a brilliant way to transform leftover cooked turkey or chicken. The trick is in the balancing of salty, sweet and sour flavours.

Hands-on time: 15 minutes, plus soaking
Cooking time: about 15 minutes
Serves 2

125g (4oz) dried flat rice
    noodles
4 tbsp Thai fish sauce
2 tbsp tamarind paste
3 tbsp demerara sugar
1 tbsp soy sauce
3 tbsp vegetable oil
2 garlic cloves, finely chopped
1 red chilli, deseeded
    and sliced
2 medium eggs, beaten
125g (4oz) cooked turkey,
    shredded
100g (3½oz) beansprouts
3 spring onions, finely sliced

TO GARNISH
2 tbsp unsalted roasted
    peanuts, roughly chopped
Small handful of fresh
    coriander, chopped
Lime wedges

**PER SERVING 704cals,
41g protein, 32g fat (5g
saturates), 62g carbs(10g
total sugars), 3g fibre**

1. Put the rice noodles in a large bowl, cover with boiling water and set aside for 5–10 minutes, or until rehydrated. Drain them and return to the bowl. Meanwhile, mix the fish sauce, tamarind, sugar, and soy sauce with 2 tablespoons water in a small pan set over a low heat. Warm them gently, stirring to dissolve the sugar. Remove from the heat and set aside.

2. Put the oil in a large frying pan or wok set over a high heat. Add the garlic and chilli, stir-fry for 30 seconds, then add the drained noodles and a splash of water and continue to stir-fry for 2 minutes more. Add the sauce and stir-fry for 1–2 minutes until the sauce is absorbed and the noodles are almost cooked through.

3. Push the noodles to one side of the wok or pan, then add the eggs to the empty section and fry, stirring, until scrambled and just set. Add the turkey, beansprouts and spring onions to the pan and stir everything together to heat through. Serve the pad thai scattered with peanuts and coriander, with lime wedges on the side to squeeze over.

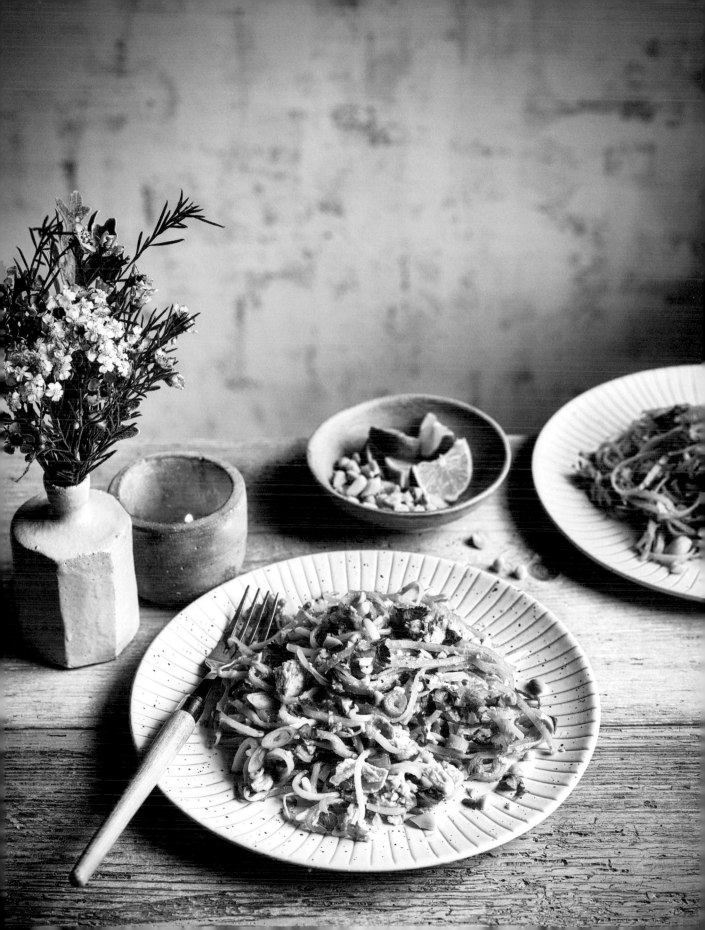

Okonomiyaki

This is our take on the Japanese savoury pancake – it's a little like the British omelette, as the filling can be adapted according to what's in your fridge. Ours uses cabbage and bacon as well as shiitake mushrooms – and that storecupboard favourite, brown sauce!

Hands-on time: 10 minutes
Cooking time: about
   20 minutes
Serves 2

150g (5oz) self-raising flour
2 medium eggs, beaten
150ml (5fl oz) cold chicken or
   vegetable stock
150g (5oz) sweetheart
   cabbage, very finely
   shredded
4 spring onions, sliced finely
1 tbsp soy sauce
1 tsp vegetable oil
125g (4oz) shiitake
   mushrooms, finely sliced
6 slices smoked streaky bacon
Pickled ginger, to serve
   (optional)
Brown sauce, to serve
   (optional)

PER SERVING 574cals,
28g protein, 22g fat (7g
saturates), 62g carbs (5g
total sugars), 7g fibre

1. Put the flour in a mixing bowl. Create a well in the centre of the flour and add the eggs, stirring gradually to create a smooth batter. Once all the egg has been incorporated, gradually add the stock. Stir through the cabbage, the white parts of the spring onions (reserve the green parts for garnish) and the soy sauce. Set aside.

2. Put the oil in a 23cm (9in) non-stick frying pan set over a medium heat and cook the mushrooms for 3–4 minutes, until golden brown and beginning to crisp. Remove with a slotted spoon and stir them through the batter mixture. Add the bacon to the pan and fry for 5 minutes until starting to crisp.

3. Spoon the batter over the bacon and gently push it with the back of the spoon to make a rough circle. Cook for 4–5 minutes until just set and golden brown on the bottom, then slide on to a plate and carefully flip so that the undercooked top side is on the bottom of the pan. Cook for a further 2–3 minutes until set on the bottom and golden brown, then transfer to a plate or board. Garnish with the remaining spring onion greens, and some pickled ginger and a drizzle of brown sauce, if you like.

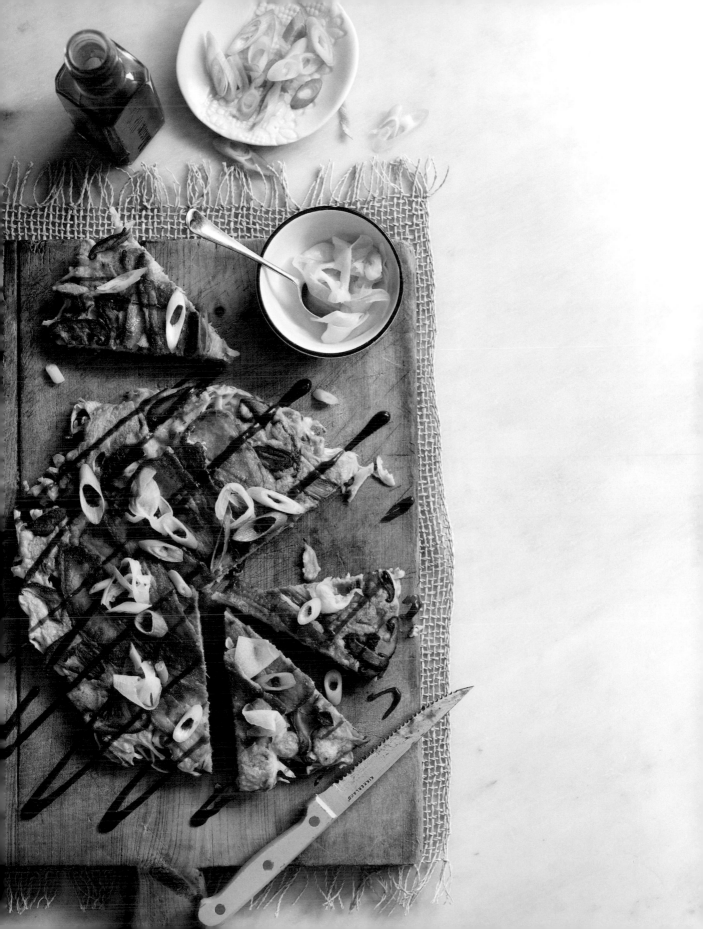

Tomato and Fennel Risotto

This recipe is easy to adapt to other vegetable combinations. If you want a meatier supper, just add some sliced cooked sausage or chicken.

Hands-on time: 15 minutes
Cooking time: about
  25 minutes
Serves 4

1 tbsp extra virgin olive oil,
  plus extra to drizzle
1 onion, finely chopped
1 fennel bulb, finely chopped
300g (11oz) risotto rice
50ml (2fl oz) white wine
400g tin tomatoes
1 tbsp tomato purée
About 800ml (1⅓ pints) hot
  gluten-free vegetable stock
40g (1½oz) vegetarian feta,
  crumbled
Large handful of fresh basil,
  roughly chopped, to garnish

PER SERVING 360cals,
9g protein, 3g fat (1g
saturates), 70g carbs (6g
total sugars), 4g fibre

1. Heat the oil in a large pan and gently fry the onion and fennel with a splash of water until softened, about 8 minutes, stirring occasionally. Increase the heat, then stir in the rice, wine, the tinned and the puréed tomatoes and cook for 1 minute.

2. Gradually add the stock, one ladleful at a time, adding each ladleful only when the previous one has been absorbed and stirring well after each addition. Continue until the rice is tender and has absorbed as much liquid as it can. This will take about 15 minutes, and use more or less stock, depending on how the rice is cooking.

3. Divide the risotto among 4 bowls and garnish with the feta, basil and a drizzle of extra virgin olive oil.

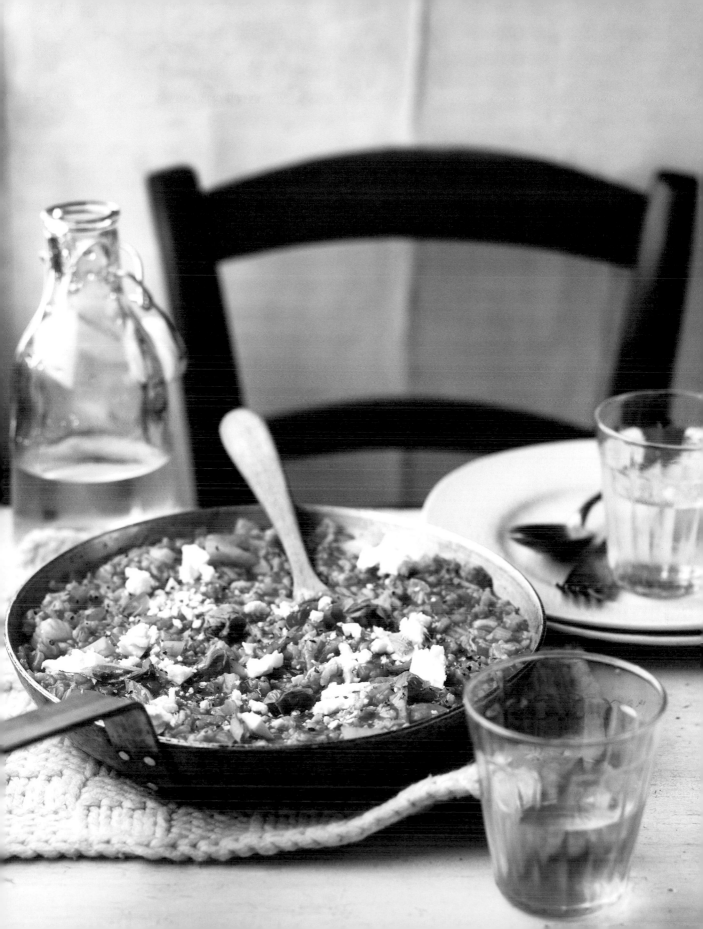

Orzo 'Paella'

Our nod to the Spanish favourite swaps traditional rice for quick-cooking orzo pasta.

Hands-on time: about 10 minutes
Cooking time: about 15 minutes
Serves 4

1 tbsp olive oil
1 onion, chopped
290g jar roasted peppers, drained and sliced
150g (5oz) cooking chorizo, sliced
2 garlic cloves, crushed
1 tbsp sweet smoked paprika
2 tbsp roasted red pepper pesto
300g (11oz) orzo pasta
250g (9oz) broad beans, shelled, if you like
Large handful fresh flat-leaf parsley, finely chopped

PER SERVING 539cals, 23g protein, 19g fat (6g saturates), 64g carbs (6g total sugars), 10g fibre

1. Heat the oil in a large frying or sauté pan (with a lid) set over a medium-high heat. Add the onion, peppers and sliced chorizo and fry for 3–4 minutes until beginning to turn golden. Add the garlic, smoked paprika and pesto and continue to cook, stirring, for 1 minute.

2. Add the orzo to the pan and cook for 1 minute, stirring constantly, to coat it in the mixture. Pour in 750ml (1¼ pints) boiling water and bring to the boil. Cover, reduce the heat to a simmer and cook gently until the liquid is mostly absorbed and the orzo is cooked, about 10 minutes.

3. Remove the lid and stir in the broad beans and parsley. Increase the heat slightly, allowing the mixture to caramelise on the bottom of the pan. Remove from the heat and serve.

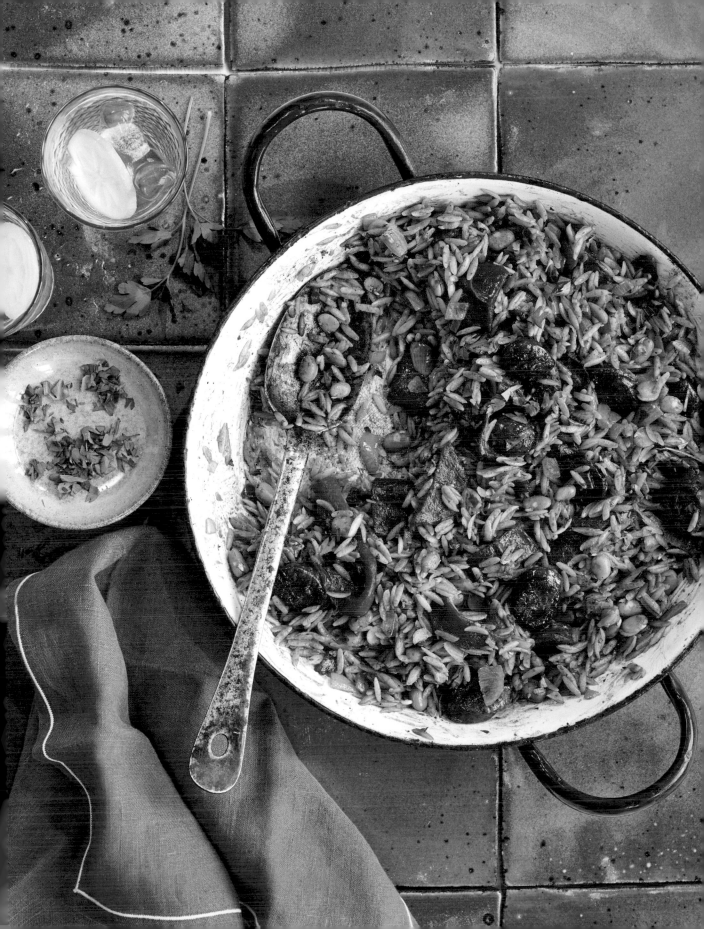

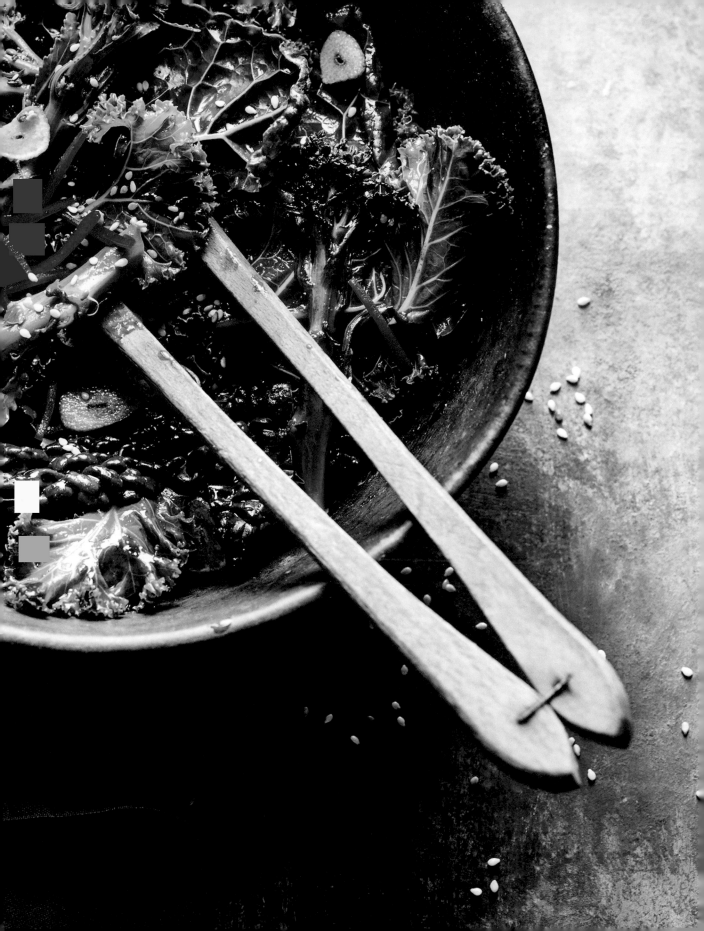

Vegetarian and Vegan

Hearty Dhal Soup with Cauliflower Rice

Warming, satisfying and very good for you, this dish is packed with veg and low in calories. Serve it with brown rice instead of cauliflower rice for a more substantial supper.

Hands-on time: 20 minutes
Cooking time: about
   25 minutes
Serves 4

1 tbsp vegetable oil
1 onion, finely chopped
2 carrots, finely chopped
2 garlic cloves, crushed
1½ tsp ground turmeric
300g (11oz) red lentils, rinsed
400g tin chopped tomatoes
1 litre (1¾ pints) gluten-free
   vegetable stock
Handful of fresh coriander,
   chopped

FOR THE CAULIFLOWER
   RICE
1 tbsp vegetable oil
2 tsp cumin seeds
2 tsp black mustard seeds
1 red chilli, deseeded and
   finely chopped
2 garlic cloves, crushed
300g (11oz) cauliflower florets

PER SERVING 370cals,
23g protein, 5g fat (1g
saturates), 53g carbs (12g
total sugars), 11g fibre

1. For the soup, heat the oil in a large pan and gently fry the onion and carrots for 5 minutes to soften. Add the garlic and turmeric and fry for a further 1 minute. Add the lentils, tomatoes and stock. Bring to the boil and simmer for 15 minutes until the lentils are tender.

2. Meanwhile, make the cauliflower rice. Heat the oil in a small frying pan. Add the cumin and mustard seeds and fry for 30 seconds until they are aromatic and the mustard seeds are beginning to pop. Add the chilli and garlic and fry for 1 minute more. Set half the spice mixture aside and add the remaining spice mix to the simmering soup.

3. Pulse the cauliflower in a food processor until it resembles rice. Heat 2 tablespoons water in a medium pan (that has a lid), then add the cauliflower and cook, covered, for 3 minutes until tender. Stir in the reserved spice mixture, season and keep warm.

4. Check the seasoning of the soup and ladle into warmed bowls. Spoon on the cauliflower rice (or serve on the side), sprinkle over the coriander and serve.

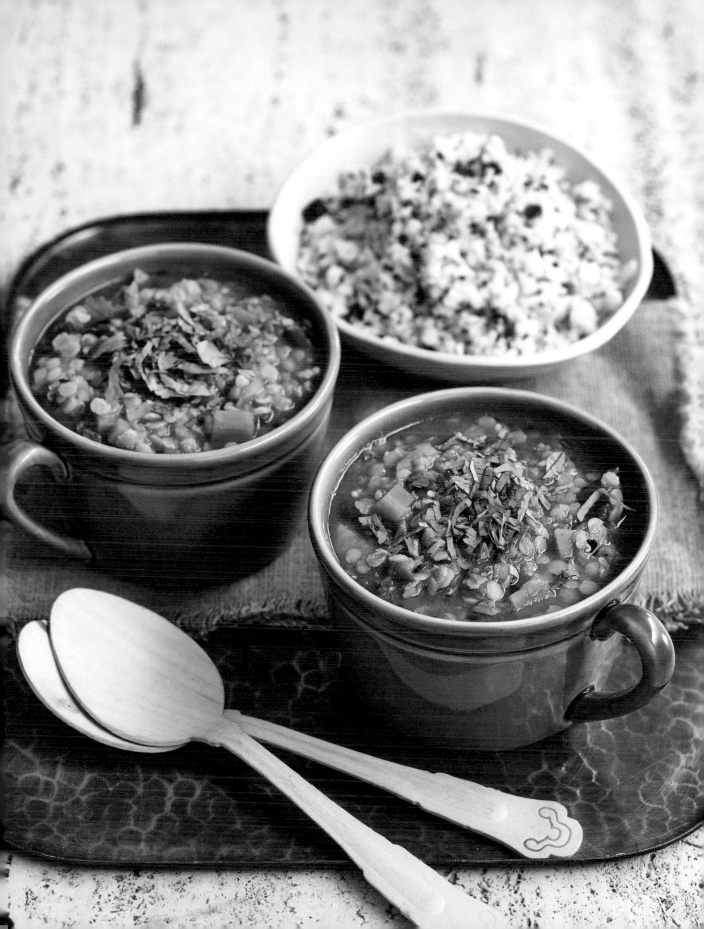

Corn, Cauliflower and Black Bean Tacos

Crunchy, creamy, punchy and zingy – these vegan-friendly tacos are full of texture and flavour.

Hands-on time: 25 minutes
Cooking time: about 10 minutes
Serves 4

2 tsp vegetable oil
2 corn on the cob
½ cauliflower, chopped into small pieces
1 tsp sweet smoked paprika
400g tin black beans, drained and rinsed
1 tbsp chipotle paste
12 soft taco shells

FOR THE SALSA AND GUACAMOLE
3 medium tomatoes, deseeded and chopped
½ small red onion, chopped
Bunch of fresh coriander, chopped
1 red chilli, finely chopped, plus extra sliced, to serve (optional)
Zest and juice of 2 limes
2 ripe avocados, de-stoned

PER SERVING 553cals, 13g protein, 33g fat (5g saturates), 46g carbs (7g total sugars), 12g fibre

1. Put the oil in a large frying pan set over high heat. Dust the corn cobs and cauliflower in the paprika. Add the corn to the hot pan and cook, turning, for about 10 minutes until charred and tender. Transfer to a plate. Add the cauliflower to the pan and stir-fry until tender and lightly charred. Stand a cob on its end on a chopping board and slice down the sides to remove the kernels. Repeat with the second cob.

2. Meanwhile, make the salsa: mix the tomatoes with the onion, coriander, chilli, the zest and juice of 1 lime and some seasoning. For the guacamole, mash the avocados with the zest and juice of the remaining lime. Add a little salt to taste. Set both aside.

3. Return the pan to the heat, add the black beans, chipotle paste and a splash of water. Cook for a few minutes, mashing some of the beans. Season to taste.

4. To serve, divide the bean mixture over the taco shells. Top with some of the charred vegetables, a spoonful of salsa and a dollop of guacamole.

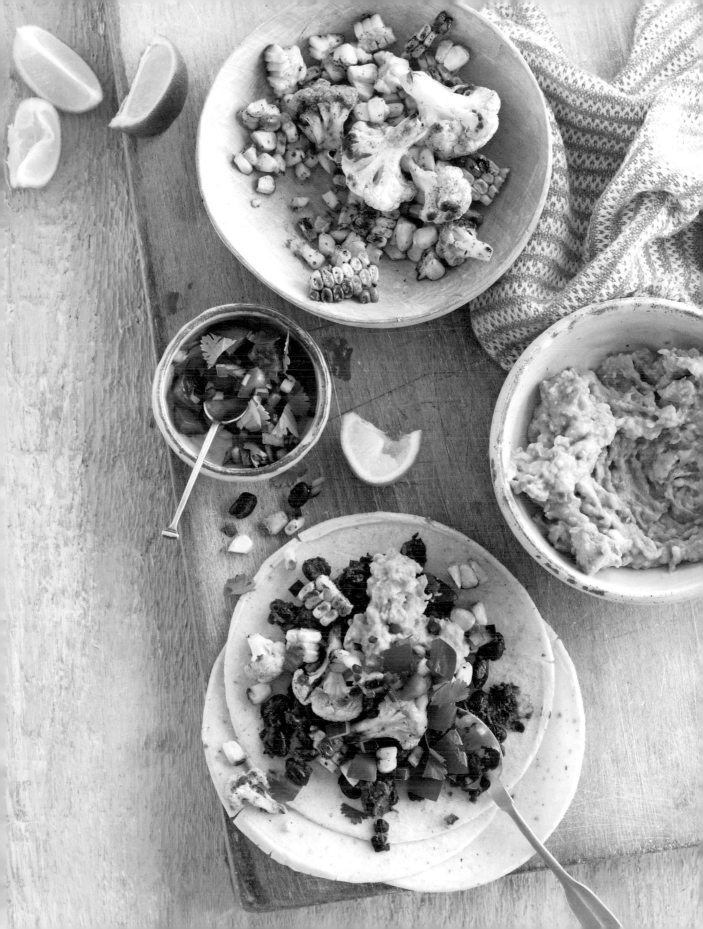

Tofu Bun Cha

This Vietnamese noodle dish is a breeze to make and packed with flavour. Desiccated coconut and panko breadcrumbs combine to make a super crispy coating for the tofu.

Hands-on time: 10 minutes
Cooking time: 10 minutes
Serves 4

396g block firm tofu
4 tbsp crunchy peanut butter
160ml tin coconut cream
1 tsp soy sauce
Juice of 1 lime
200g (7oz) dried flat rice
    noodles
1 small cucumber
2 carrots
1 tbsp sesame oil
3 tbsp vegetable oil
3 tbsp cornflour, seasoned
4 tbsp panko breadcrumbs
2 tbsp desiccated coconut
Small handful each of fresh
    mint and coriander
1 red chilli, sliced
2 tbsp dry roasted peanuts,
    crushed

**PER SERVING 864cals,
30g protein, 50g fat (17g
saturates), 70g carbs (8g
total sugars), 9g fibre**

1. Cut the tofu into 12 slices and leave to dry on kitchen paper to soak up any excess liquid.

2. To make the dressing, whisk together the peanut butter, coconut cream, soy sauce and lime juice in a bowl. Whisk in a little hot water to loosen, if you like. Season to taste.

3. Cook the rice noodles according to the pack instructions, then drain, run under cold water, drain again and put into a large bowl. Using a spiralizer or peeler, grate the cucumber (discard the seedy middle) and carrots into the noodle bowl. Drizzle over the sesame oil and toss gently through the ingredients, then cover and set aside.

4. Put the vegetable oil in a frying pan set over medium-high heat. Fill a small bowl with cornflour, another with cold water and a final bowl with the panko crumbs and coconut. Dip each piece of tofu into the cornflour, then the water and finally into the crumb mixture to coat. Cook the tofu in the oil for 2–3 minutes until golden and crisp.

5. Divide the vegetable noodles and most of the herbs among 4 bowls, top with the hot tofu, drizzle with half the peanut sauce and garnish with the chilli, crushed peanuts and remaining herbs. Serve with the remaining peanut sauce on the side.

◆ GET AHEAD
Make the peanut sauce a day ahead and keep it covered in the fridge. Bring to room temperature before serving.

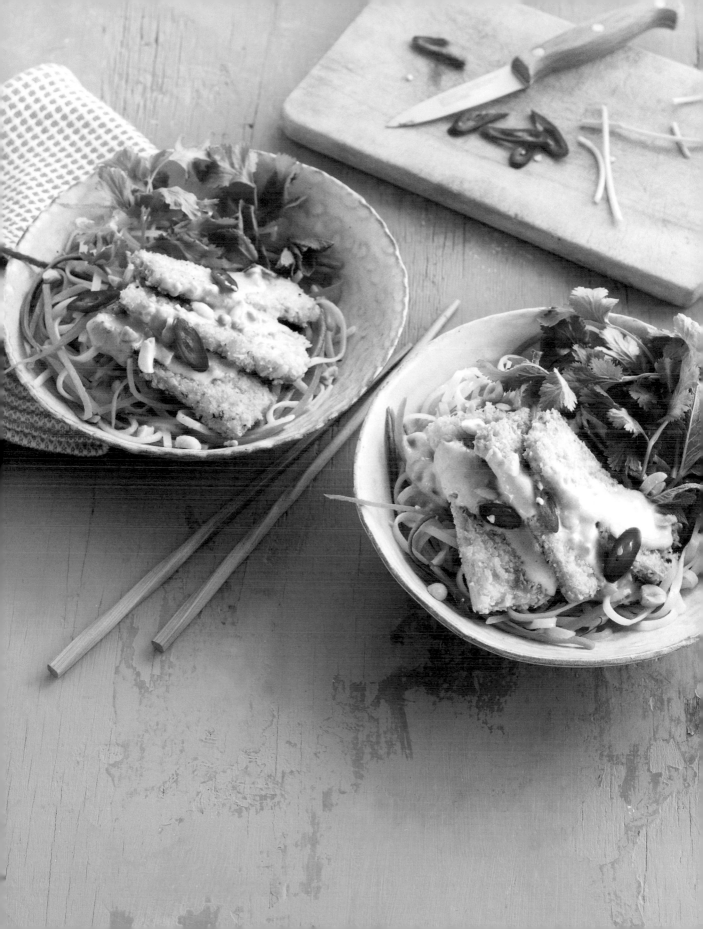

Lentil Niçoise

We've given classic Tuna Niçoise a vegetarian makeover by swapping the fish for protein-rich puy lentils. There's so much flavour in the sprightly dressing, piquant olives and soft-boiled eggs that you won't miss the tuna.

Hands-on time: 10 minutes
Cooking time: 15 minutes
Serves 4

4 medium eggs, at room
    temperature
200g (7oz) fine green beans
2 x 250g pouches ready-
    cooked puy lentils
100g (3½oz) pitted black
    olives, chopped
150g (5oz) mixed radishes,
    sliced

FOR THE DRESSING
1 shallot, finely chopped
1 tsp Dijon mustard
5 tbsp extra virgin olive oil
1½ tbsp white wine vinegar
Small bunch of fresh flat-leaf
    parsley, finely chopped

PER SERVING 422cals,
21g protein, 24g fat (4g
saturates), 25g carbs (3g
total sugars), 12g fibre

1. Add the eggs to a small pan of salted simmering water and cook for 8 minutes. Meanwhile, in a small bowl, whisk all the dressing ingredients together and season. Set aside.

2. Remove the eggs with a slotted spoon (keeping the pan of water on the heat) and transfer to a bowl of ice-cold water to prevent further cooking. Leave the eggs to cool for 5 minutes, then drain. Peel the eggs and cut in half.

3. Bring the pan of water back to the boil, add the beans and cook for 3–4 minutes until al dente. Drain and transfer into a bowl of ice-cold water to cool quickly, then drain again.

4. In a large bowl, toss the beans and lentils with half of the dressing. Tip on to a platter, scatter over the olives, radishes and halved eggs. Drizzle over the remaining dressing and serve straight away.

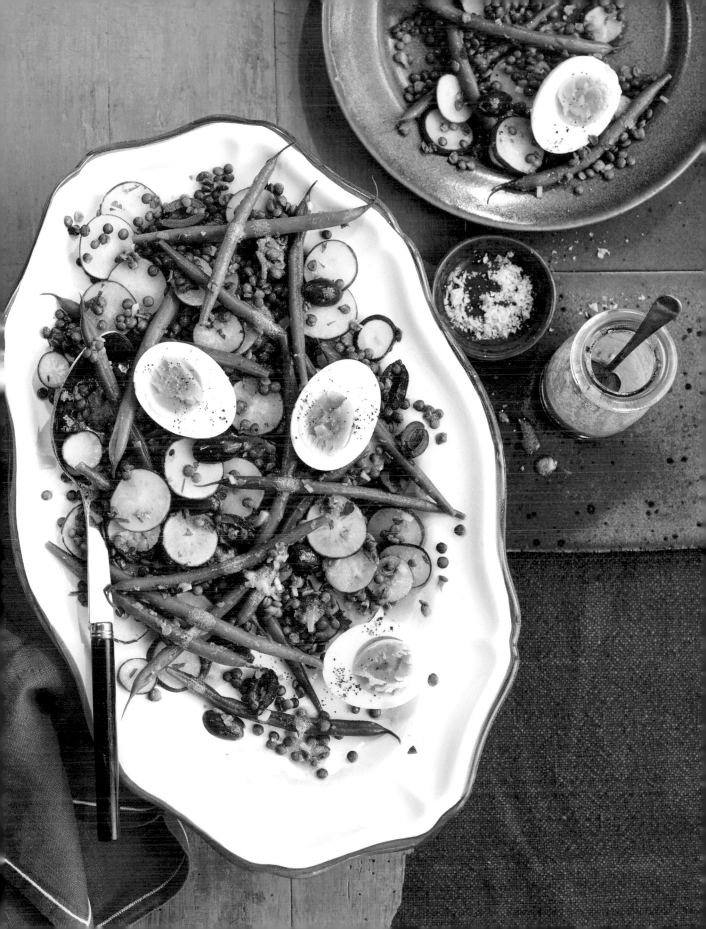

Fig and Fennel Grain Salad

Rich, nutty spelt is packed with protein and fibre to help you feel full for longer. Serve this as a main course, a side dish, or packed into a lunchbox for meals on the go.

Hands-on time: 10 minutes
Cooking time: 20 minutes
Serves 6

2 fennel bulbs, cut into
    wedges
3 tbsp olive oil
2 oranges
1 tbsp sherry vinegar
2 x 250g ready-cooked mixed
    grain pouches (we used a
    mix of spelt, brown rice and
    barley)
60g bag rocket
1 radicchio, shredded
3 fresh figs, quartered
2 tbsp mixed seeds

PER SERVING 260cals,
7g protein, 10g fat (1g
saturates), 32g carbs (8g
total sugars), 8g fibre

1. Heat a griddle pan to medium hot. Brush the fennel wedges with a little of the oil and cook for 4–5 minutes on each side. Set aside and keep warm.

2. To make the dressing, carefully peel and segment the orange over a bowl to catch the juice. Put the segments in a separate bowl. Whisk the remaining oil and vinegar into the orange juice and season to taste.

3. Heat the grains according to the pack instructions, then tip into a large bowl and pour over 4 tablespoons of the dressing. Stir well with a fork to break down any chunks of grain and allow the grains to cool slightly.

4. Stir the orange segments, rocket and radicchio through the grains and spoon the salad on to a platter. Top with the fennel wedges, figs, mixed seeds and remaining dressing. Serve.

◆ GET AHEAD
Make the salad up to 3 hours before serving, leaving out the rocket and radicchio. Cover and chill. Bring back to room temperature and stir through the fresh leaves when you're ready to serve.

Aubergine and Chickpea Masala

This delicious, filling curry will please veggies and meat-eaters alike.

Hands-on time: 15 minutes
Cooking time: about 25 minutes
Serves 4

1½ tbsp oil
1 large onion, thinly sliced
1 aubergine, cut into 2cm (¾in) chunks
4 medium potatoes, cut into 2cm (¾in) chunks
3 tbsp mild curry paste
1 tsp black mustard seeds
350ml (12fl oz) gluten-free vegetable stock
250g (9oz) basmati rice, washed
400g tin chickpeas, drained and rinsed
3 tbsp mango chutney
Large handful of fresh coriander leaves, roughly chopped, plus extra to garnish
Natural yogurt, to serve

PER SERVING 547cals, 16g protein, 10g fat (0.8g saturates), 94g carbs (10g total sugars), 9g fibre

1. Put the oil in a large pan set over medium heat. Add the onion and cook for 5 minutes until softened. Turn up the heat, add the aubergine and potatoes, then fry for 5 minutes more, stirring frequently so the mixture doesn't catch.

2. Stir in the curry paste and mustard seeds and fry for 30 seconds. Add the stock and simmer, covered, for 15 minutes (stirring occasionally) until the vegetables are tender.

3. Meanwhile, cook the rice in boiling salted water for 12–15 minutes or until tender. Drain well and keep warm.

4. Stir the chickpeas, chutney and coriander into the curry, then check the seasoning. Serve with the boiled rice and a dollop of natural yogurt, garnished with extra coriander leaves.

Charred Broccoli, Butterbeans and Romesco on Toast

A smoky, almond-rich romesco sauce really livens up simple veg on toast. This dish is ideal for brunch or lunch.

Hands-on time: 15 minutes
Cooking time: 10 minutes
Serves 4

175g (6oz) roasted red peppers
    in brine, drained
50g (2oz) toasted flaked
    almonds
1 tsp sweet smoked paprika
1 small garlic clove, crushed
4 tbsp olive oil, plus extra
    to toss
215g tin butterbeans, drained
    and rinsed
300g (11oz) Tenderstem
    broccoli, trimmed
8 spring onions, trimmed
4 slices seeded sourdough
    bread
2 tbsp chopped fresh parsley

PER SERVING 393cals,
15g protein, 19g fat (2g
saturates), 36g carbs (4g
total sugars), 10g fibre

1. Roughly chop the roasted peppers and tip into a small food processor with the almonds, paprika, garlic and 2 tablespoons olive oil. Whiz to a chunky sauce, season to taste, then tip into a bowl. Cover and set aside until needed.

2. Tip the butterbeans into the processor and whiz with 2 tablespoons oil and 1 teaspoon boiling water until smooth. Season, cover and set aside.

3. Toss the broccoli and spring onions in a little oil. Heat a griddle pan to medium high and cook them for 2–3 minutes on each side until lightly charred.

4. Toast the bread, spread with bean purée and top with the charred vegetables. Spoon over the sauce and sprinkle over the parsley to serve.

● GH TIP
Try the romesco sauce as a dip with crudités or pitta crisps.

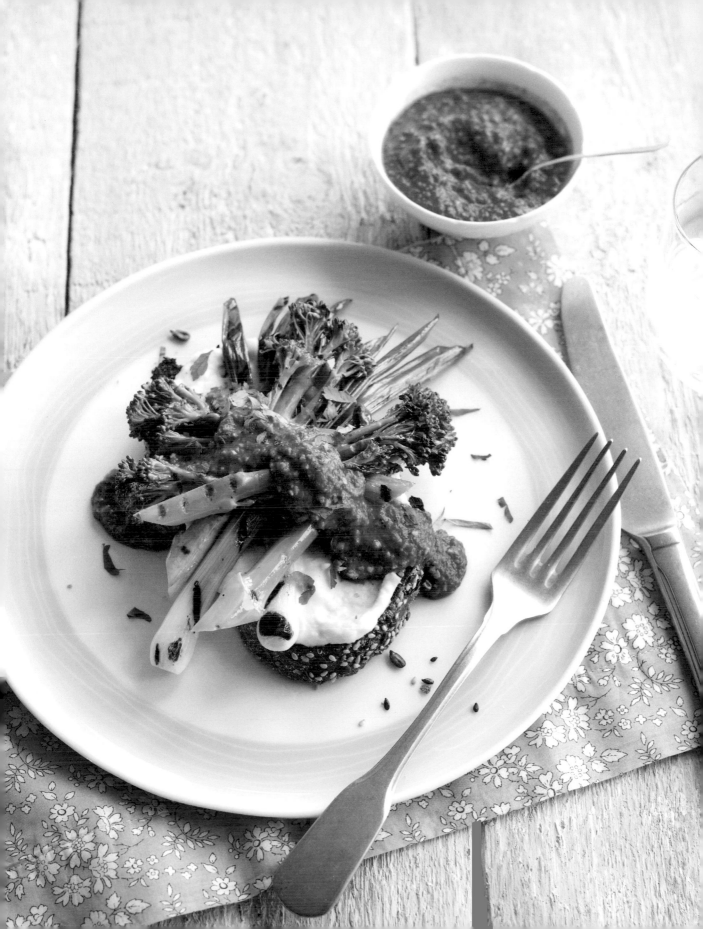

Mushroom, Kale and Walnut Pesto Linguine

Honey adds a lovely sweetness to balance the earthiness of the kale in this recipe – add more to taste, if you like.

Hands-on time: 10 minutes
Cooking time: 15 minutes
Serves 4

75g (3oz) kale, washed
25g (1oz) shelled walnuts
3 tbsp olive oil, plus extra to
   drizzle
25g (1oz) grated Parmesan-
   style vegetarian hard
   cheese, plus extra to garnish
½ tbsp lemon juice
½ tbsp clear honey
300g (11oz) linguine
250g (9oz) mushrooms, sliced
1 garlic clove, crushed

PER SERVING 443cals,
16g protein, 17g fat (3g
saturates), 55g carbs (4g
total sugars), 5g fibre

1. Put the kale, walnuts, 2 tablespoons of the olive oil, cheese, lemon juice and honey into a food processor. Pulse until smooth and season to taste.

2. Meanwhile, bring a large pan of salted water to the boil and cook the linguine according to the pack instructions.

3. Heat the remaining oil in a pan and fry the mushrooms and garlic together until golden and cooked through.

4. Drain the pasta, then stir through pesto and mushrooms. Add a drizzle of olive oil and sprinkle with extra cheese.

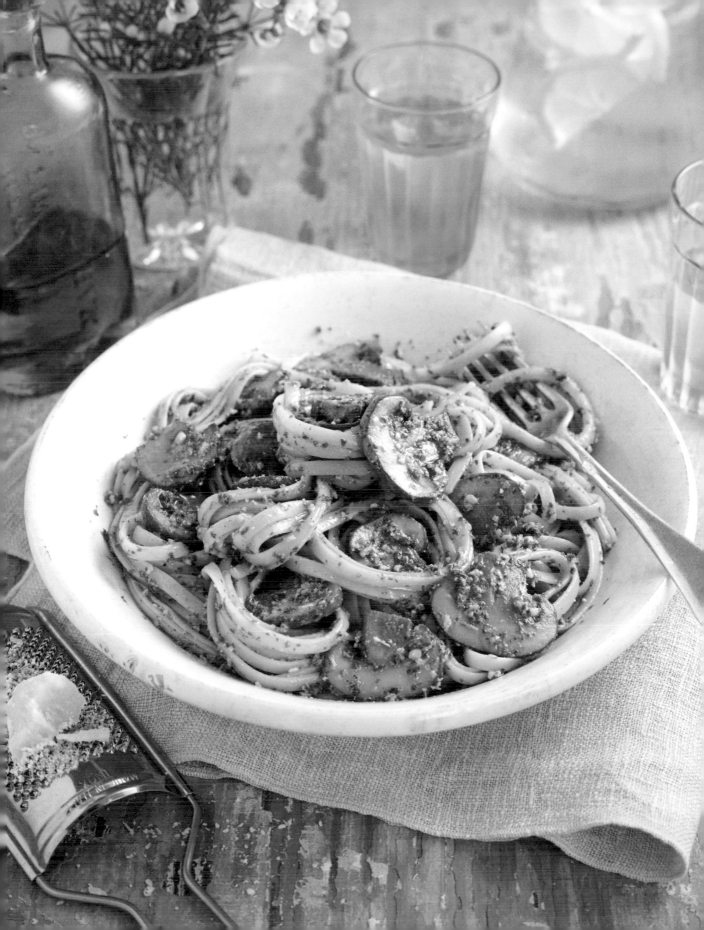

Tofu Pad Thai

Pressing the tofu before you fry it is a worthwhile step, as it develops a firmer texture when drier.

Hands-on time: 20 minutes, plus pressing.
Cooking time: about 10 minutes
Serves 4

396g block firm tofu (not silken)
1 tbsp sunflower oil
300g (11oz) dried flat rice noodles
1 red pepper, deseeded and sliced
1 garlic clove, finely chopped
3 tbsp soy sauce
1 tbsp vegan Thai fish sauce
3 spring onions, sliced
Juice of 1 lime
40g (1½oz) salted peanuts, roughly chopped

PER SERVING 483cals, 21g protein, 15g fat (1g saturates), 64g carbs (4g total sugars), 4g fibre

1. Drain and dry the tofu well with kitchen paper. Sit the tofu block on a baking tray lined with kitchen paper. Cover the tofu with more kitchen paper and another baking tray, then set a heavy pan on top. Leave to press for 15 minutes, then cut the tofu into 2.5cm (1in) cubes.

2. Put half the oil in a large non-stick frying pan or wok set over high heat and fry the tofu, turning gently, to brown it on all sides. Carefully lift out of the pan on to a plate and set aside.

3. Meanwhile, cook the rice noodles according to the pack instructions, then drain. Run them under cold water to stop them cooking further, then drain again.

4. Return the empty frying pan or wok to high heat with the remaining oil. Stir-fry the pepper for 1 minute, then stir in the garlic, cooked noodles and soy and fish sauces to heat through. Carefully fold through the tofu, spring onions and lime juice. Check the seasoning and serve immediately, sprinkled with peanuts.

● GH TIP
Vegetarian and vegan Thai 'fish' sauce is now widely available at larger supermarkets. Use tamari instead of soy sauce to make this dish gluten free.

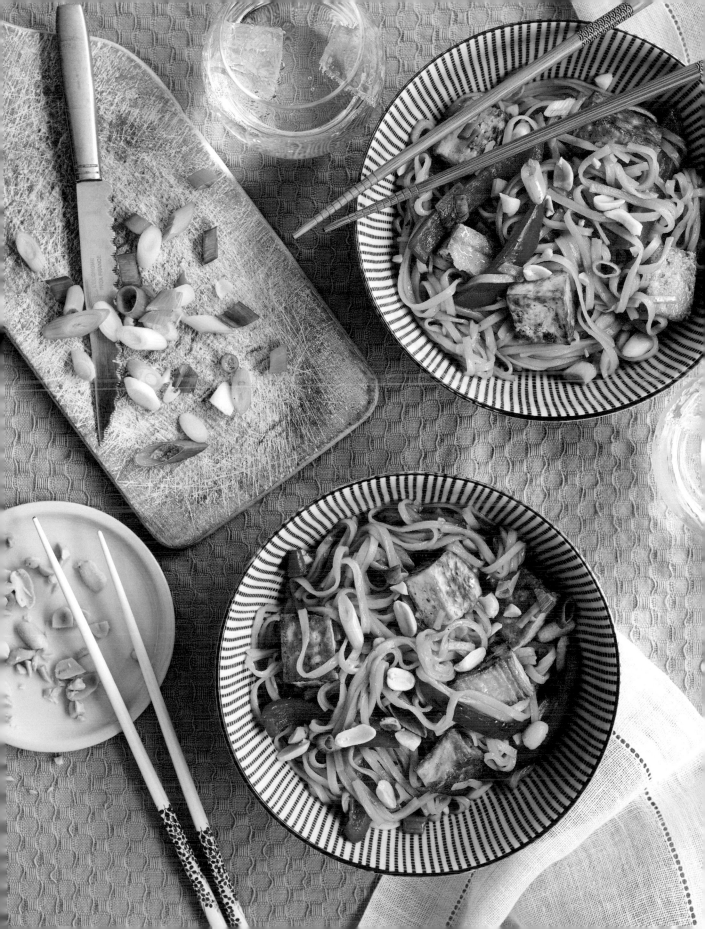

Spiced Paneer Burrito

Paneer is a firm Indian cheese with a mild flavour that takes on spices beautifully.

Hands-on time: 10 minutes
Cooking time: 5 minutes
Serves 4

226g pack paneer cheese
2 tbsp tikka masala curry
  paste
2 x 250g pouches ready-
  cooked pilau rice
4 large flour tortilla wraps
150g (5oz) natural yogurt
Large bunch of fresh
  coriander, chopped
2 fresh mint sprigs, leaves
  chopped
100g (3½oz) baby spinach
4 heaped tbsp mango chutney

PER SERVING 606cals,
22g protein, 20g fat (10g
saturates), 83g carbs (17g
total sugars), 4g fibre

1. Cut the paneer into strips and put in a bowl with the curry paste and some seasoning. Toss gently to coat in the spice paste.

2. Set a large non-stick frying pan over high heat. Add the seasoned paneer strips to the pan in a single layer and fry for a couple of minutes on each side until golden.

3. Meanwhile, heat the rice according to the pack instructions.

4. Bring the paneer, wraps, rice, yogurt, herbs, spinach and mango chutney on separate plates or in small bowls to the table and let people assemble their burritos themselves.

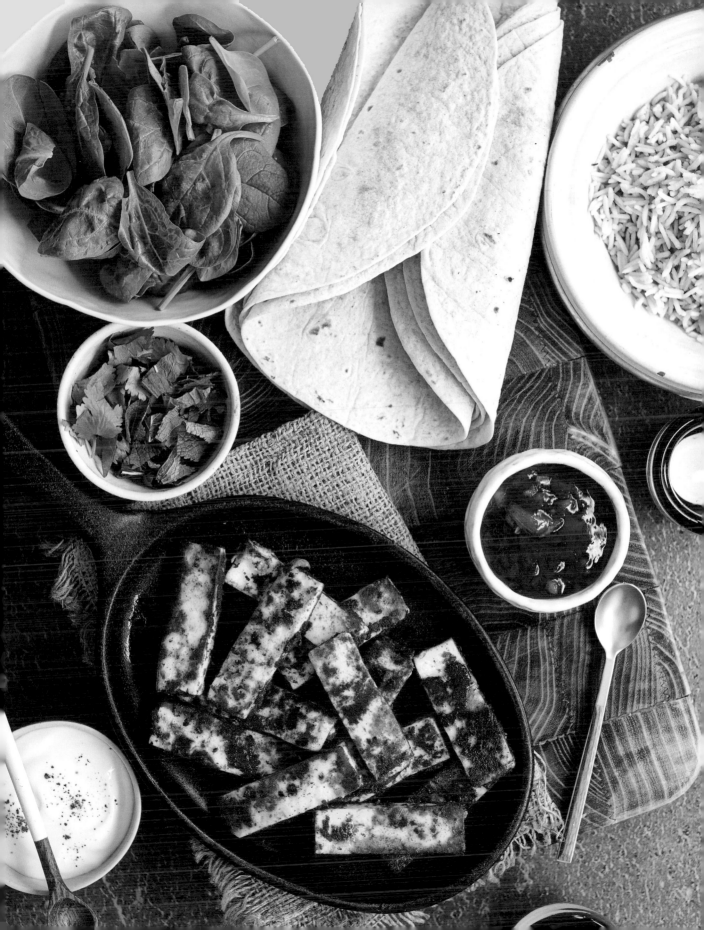

Halloumi, Watermelon and Grains Salad

Refreshing and sweet, watermelon goes beautifully with salty halloumi and fragrant mint. We've used ready-cooked grains in this recipe – choose a gluten-free variety, if you like.

Hands-on time: 15 minutes
Cooking time: about
   5 minutes
Serves 2

250g pouch ready-cooked
   grains
6 slices halloumi (about
   180g/6oz)
½ cucumber, deseeded and
   cut into half-moons
450g (1lb) prepared
   watermelon, cut into 2–3cm
   (¾–1¼in) chunks
Large handful of fresh mint,
   leaves picked and roughly
   chopped, plus a few extra
   leaves to garnish

FOR THE DRESSING
2 tbsp olive oil
½ tsp each bruised coriander
   and cumin seeds
2 tbsp freshly squeezed
   orange juice
½ tbsp sherry vinegar
½ tbsp runny honey

PER SERVING 688cals,
30g protein, 37g fat (18g
saturates), 55g carbs (22g
total sugars), 8g fibre

1. For the dressing, gently heat the olive oil in a frying pan and toast the spices for 5 minutes, until fragrant. Remove from the heat, then whisk in the orange juice, vinegar and honey. Allow to cool, then season to taste. Set aside.

2. Heat the grains according to the pack instructions and set aside to cool slightly.

3. Set a non-stick frying pan over medium-high heat. Cook the halloumi slices for 1–2 minutes on each side until golden brown.

4. Meanwhile, tip the grains into a large bowl, add the cucumber, watermelon, most of the dressing and the mint. Toss together. Pile on to a platter and top with the cooked halloumi, remaining dressing and mint.

● GH TIP
Swap the halloumi for vegetarian feta, or serve with barbecued lamb for any meat eaters.

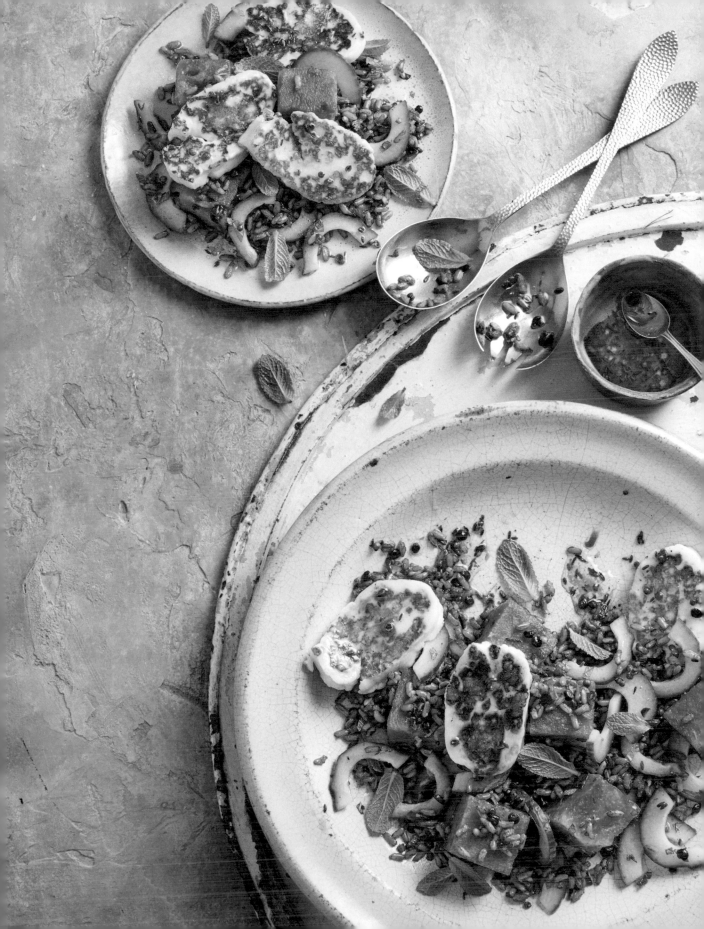

Gyoza and Spiralized Veg Bowl

Japanese miso paste (made from fermented soya beans and rice, barley, wheat or rye) is a handy fridge staple and provides an instant depth of flavour in soups like this one. You can also use it as a glaze for grilled meat, fish or aubergines, or in dressings and marinades.

Hands-on time: 10 minutes
Cooking time: about
**   20 minutes**
Serves 2

1 bunch (about 6) spring
    onions
1 litre (1¾ pints) hot vegan
    vegetable stock
1 red chilli, sliced
Small bunch of fresh
    coriander, leaves and stalks
    chopped separately
3 tbsp white miso paste
1 tbsp soy sauce, plus extra
    to serve
16 frozen vegan vegetable
    gyoza, taken from a 300g
    bag
125g (4oz) frozen soya beans
300g (11oz) spiralized
    courgette

PER SERVING 464cals,
29g protein, 13g fat (1g
saturates), 53g carbs (14g
total sugars), 11g fibre

1. Finely chop the white part of the spring onions and add to a large pan with the stock, half the chilli and the chopped coriander stalks. Bring to the boil, then lower the heat and simmer gently for 5 minutes.

2. Meanwhile, finely slice the green tops of the onion lengthways into long thin strips and put in a bowl of iced water so they go curly. Set aside until ready to serve.

3. After 5 minutes, stir the miso paste into the stock until dissolved, then add the soy sauce. Add the gyoza and soya beans to the stock and bring back to the boil, cook for 1 minute, then add the spiralized courgette and cook for a further 1-2 minutes until tender. Ladle into 2 bowls, top with coriander leaves, the drained spring onion greens and the remaining chilli.

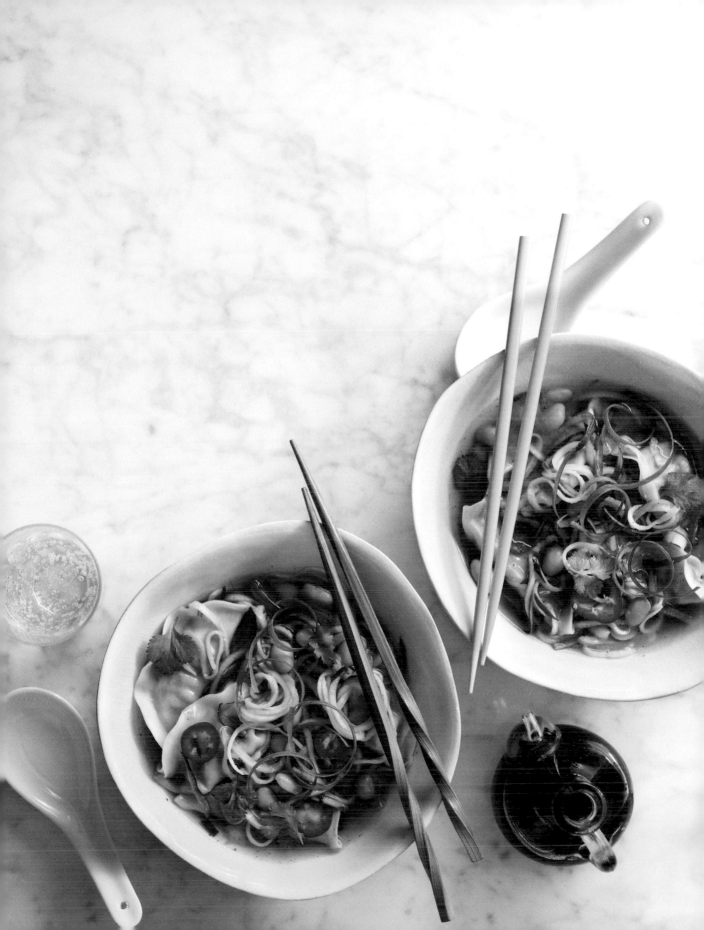

Korean Stir-fried Greens

Pep up winter greens with punchy Asian flavours in this stir-fried side dish. It's delicious alongside grilled mushrooms, tofu or fish (for non-vegetarians). Gochugang is a Korean chilli paste available in most large supermarkets.

Hands-on time: 10 minutes
Cooking time: about 10 minutes
Serves 4

1 tbsp gochujang Korean spice paste
1 tbsp soy sauce
1 tbsp rice wine vinegar
1 tbsp runny honey
1 tbsp sunflower oil
1 garlic clove, finely sliced
500g (1lb 2oz) mixed greens (such as whole leaf kale, cavolo nero and purple sprouting broccoli)
1 tsp sesame oil
½ red chilli, finely sliced
Pinch of toasted sesame seeds

PER SERVING 101cals,
4g protein, 5g fat (1g saturates), 7g carbs (7g total sugars), 6g fibre

1. In a small bowl, mix together the spice paste, soy sauce, rice wine vinegar and runny honey. Set aside

2. Put the oil in a wok set over medium heat, then add the garlic and stir-fry until it turns golden. Add the mixed greens and increase the heat to high. Stir-fry for a few minutes more, then add the spice mixture and toss the ingredients together to coat in the sauce. Cook for a further few minutes until the greens are just tender. Remove from the heat, stir in the sesame oil and sprinkle over the chilli and sesame seeds. Serve straightaway.

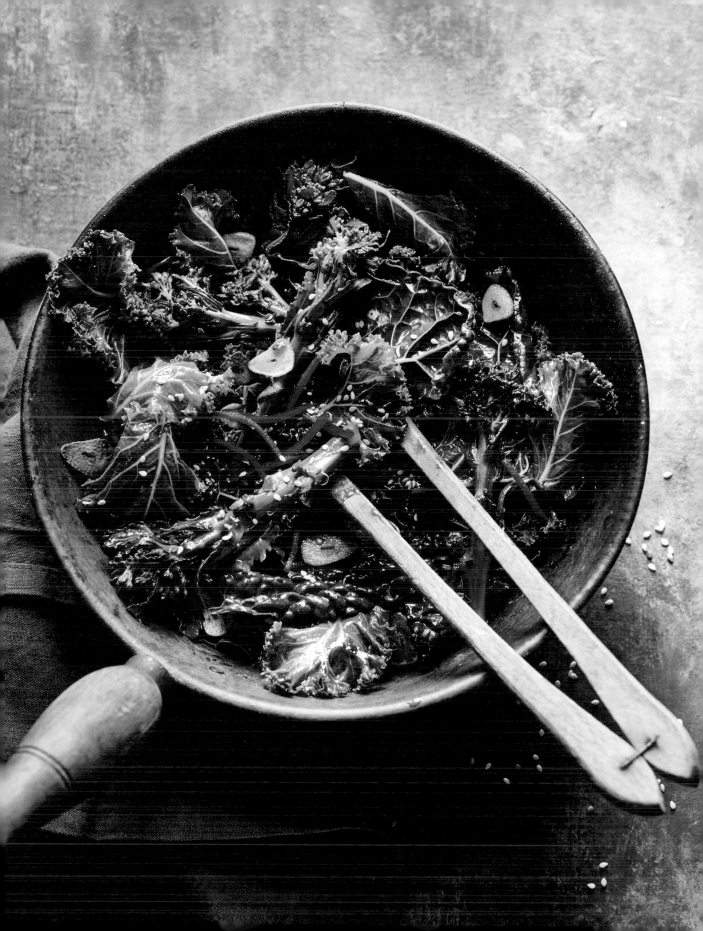

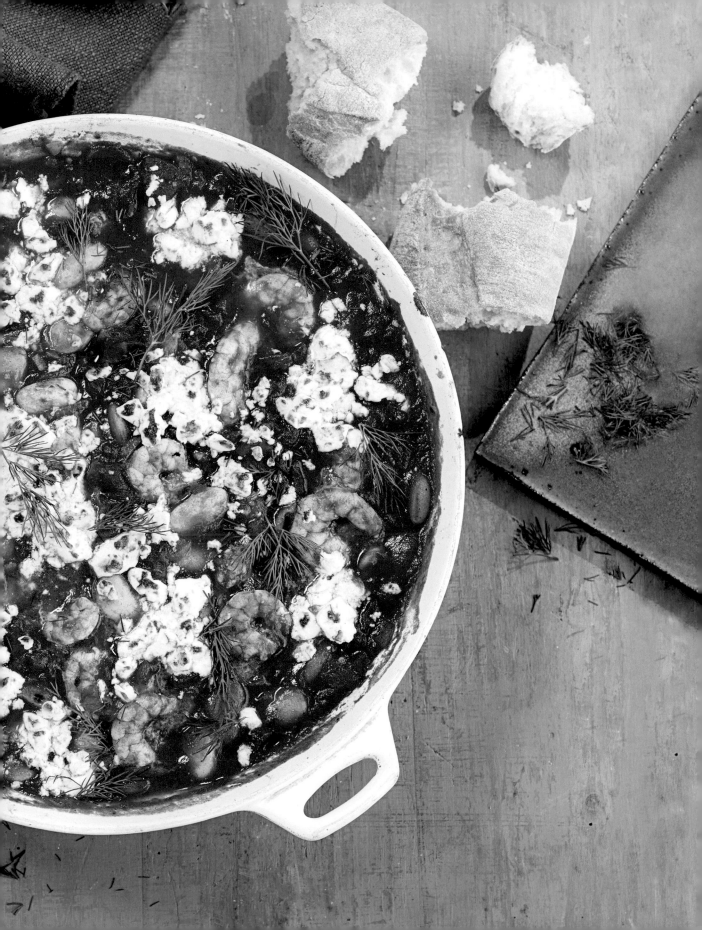

Lighten Up
Under 500 Calories

Chicken Pozole

A Mexican soup or stew, pozole is traditionally made with hominy – corn kernels that have been soaked in a mineral lime solution. Hominy can be difficult to find in shops, so we've substituted chickpeas, which work equally well and are a storecupboard staple.

Hands-on time: 20 minutes
Cooking time: about
   10 minutes
Serves 4

1 tbsp vegetable oil
325g (11½oz) skinless and
   boneless chicken thigh
   fillets, cut into bite-sized
   pieces
2 garlic cloves, crushed
2 tsp ground cumin
1½ tbsp chopped fresh
   oregano (or use 1 tsp dried)
1–2 green chillies, to taste,
   deseeded and finely chopped
1 litre (1¾ pints) gluten-free,
   strong chicken stock
2 plum tomatoes, chopped
2 x 400g tins chickpeas,
   drained and rinsed

TO SERVE
½ iceberg lettuce, shredded
Lime wedges
6 radishes, finely sliced
½ red onion, finely sliced
1 avocado, stoned and sliced
Large handful of fresh
   coriander, roughly chopped

**PER SERVING 439cals,
31g protein, 22g fat (5g
saturates), 24g carbs (4g
total sugars), 11g fibre**

1. Put the oil in a large, deep frying pan set over a medium-high heat. Add the chicken and fry until lightly golden (it doesn't need to be cooked through at this stage). Stir in the garlic, cumin, oregano and chillies, then fry for 1 minute until aromatic.

2. Pour the stock into the pan and bring to the boil. Add the tomatoes and chickpeas, then simmer for a couple of minutes until the tomatoes begin to break down. Check the seasoning. Ladle into 4 bowls and bring to the table with the garnishes in small bowls. Let people customise their stew by adding what they like before they tuck in.

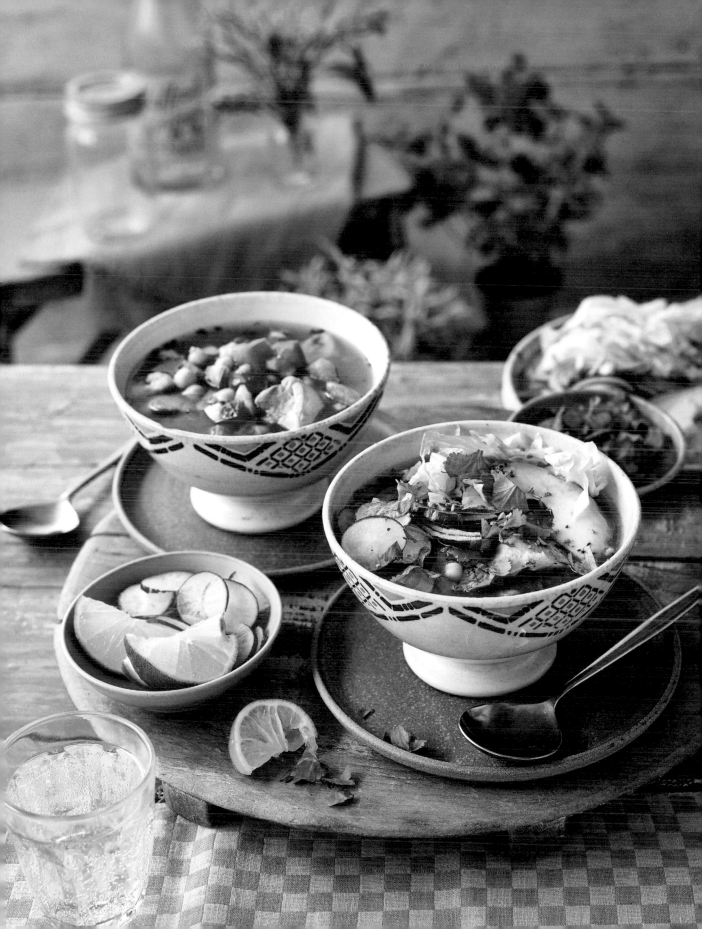

Smoked Mackerel Kedgeree

We've adapted this brunch favourite to make a healthy-yet-hearty midweek meal. Rich in omega-3s and high in fibre, thanks to the oily fish and brown rice, this flavour-packed supper will keep you feeling full for longer, and is gluten free, too. Using ready-cooked rice makes this speedy to prepare.

Hands-on time: 10 minutes
Cooking time: about
   20 minutes
Serves 4

1 tbsp olive oil
1 onion, finely sliced
1 tbsp gluten-free medium
   curry powder
¼ tsp ground turmeric
2 x 250g pouches ready-
   cooked wholegrain rice
200ml (⅓ pint) hot gluten-free
   vegetable stock
2 large eggs
225g (8oz) smoked peppered
   mackerel
2 tomatoes, finely chopped
Juice of 1 lemon, plus extra
   wedges to serve (optional)
Handful of fresh parsley,
   roughly chopped

PER SERVING 479cals,
22g protein, 23g fat (5g
saturates), 44g carbs (4g
total sugars), 5g fibre

1. Heat the oil in a large, deep frying pan. Gently fry the onion for 8–10 minutes until soft. Add the spices and cook for 1 minute. Stir in the rice to coat it in the spicy oil and fry for 1 minute. Add the stock, then bring up to the boil and simmer for 3–5 minutes until piping hot.

2. Meanwhile, bring a medium pan of water to the boil, add the eggs and simmer for 7 minutes to soft boil or a minute longer if you prefer them set. Drain the eggs into a colander and run them under cold water until they feel cold, then peel and halve. Flake the mackerel, discarding any skin.

3. Mix the tomatoes, lemon juice and parsley with the rice mixture and season well. Transfer to a serving platter, then top with the mackerel and eggs. Serve with extra lemon wedges to squeeze over, if you like.

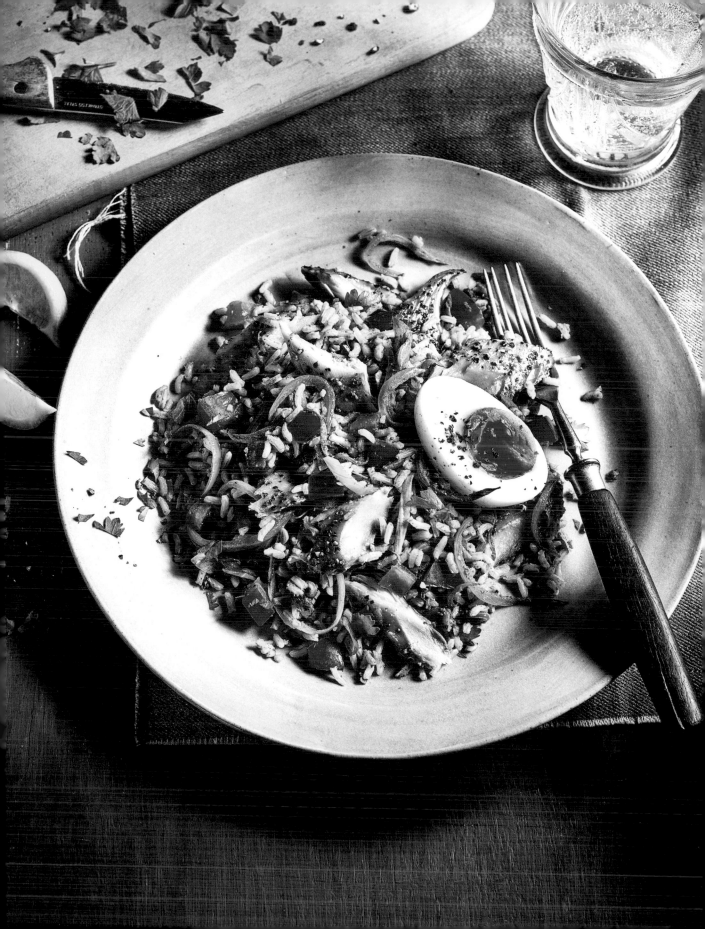

Ham Hock, Jersey Royal and Broad Bean Salad

Jersey Royals are only available in the Spring for a short time – if you're making this at a different time of year, simply use any variety of new potatoes you can find.

Hands-on time: 10 minutes
Cooking time: 10 minutes
Serves 4

500g (1lb 2oz) Jersey Royal or
  other new potatoes, halved
  if large
1 tsp olive oil
100g (3½oz) broad beans,
  fresh or frozen
100g (3½oz) sugar snap peas
125g (4oz) lamb's lettuce or
  watercress
50g (2oz) mixed radishes,
  sliced
About 200g (7oz) cooked
  pulled ham hock
5 tbsp natural yogurt
1 tsp English mustard
3 tbsp chopped fresh tarragon

PER SERVING 219cals,
17g protein, 4g fat (1g
saturates), 25g carbs (5g
total sugars), 6g fibre

1. Add the potatoes to a pan of salted cold water, then bring to the boil and simmer for 10–12 minutes until just tender. Drain, toss in the oil and set aside to cool.

2. Meanwhile, cook the broad beans and sugar snaps for 1–2 minutes in salted boiling water. Drain and plunge them into a bowl of cold water.

3. Toss the lamb's lettuce or watercress and the radishes together on a large serving plate, then top with the potatoes, broad beans, sugar snaps and ham.

4. To make the dressing, stir together the yogurt, mustard and tarragon with plenty of black pepper and season with salt to taste. Drizzle over the salad and serve straight away.

● GH TIP
Swap the ham for poached salmon or smoked mackerel, if you prefer

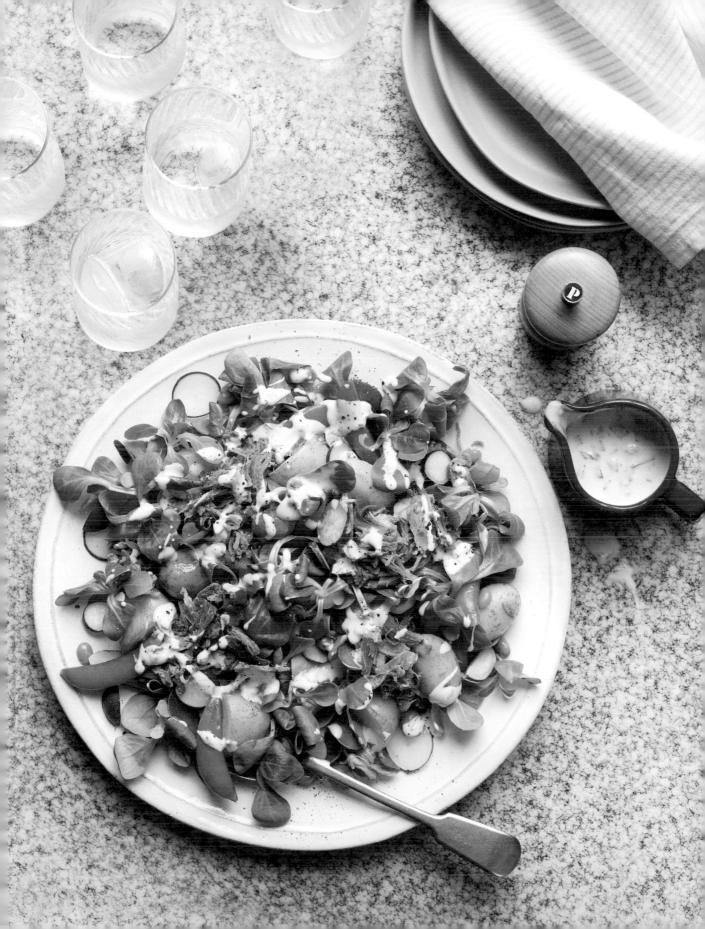

Take-to-work Sushi Salmon Salad

Make this salad the night before and you'll have a delicious, nutritious and filling lunch to enjoy the next day.

Hands-on time: 10 minutes, plus pickling
Serves 2

50g (2oz) soya beans, defrosted if frozen
¼ cucumber, peeled into ribbons
100g (3½oz) radishes, sliced
2½ tbsp rice vinegar
1 tsp caster sugar
1 tsp toasted sesame oil
250g pouch ready-cooked wholegrain rice
Zest and juice of 1 lime
Pinch of dried chilli flakes
1 tbsp soy sauce
1 tsp runny honey
2 tbsp pickled ginger
2 hot smoked or poached salmon fillets
½ tsp each black and white sesame seeds

Per serving 435cals,
32g protein, 13g fat (2g saturates), 46g carbs (9g total sugars), 4g fibre

1. In a bowl, mix together the soya beans, cucumber, radishes, 1 tablespoon rice vinegar and a pinch of salt. Set aside for 10 minutes to pickle.

2. Meanwhile, in a small bowl, whisk together the sugar, remaining rice vinegar, sesame oil and a pinch of salt. Stir through the rice.

3. For the dressing, whisk together the lime zest and juice, chilli flakes, soy sauce and honey. Decant the dressing into a small jar or pot if you plan to take the salad with you the next day.

4. Divide the rice between 2 lunchboxes, then top each with a pile of the pickled veg, a little pickled ginger, a flaked salmon fillet and a sprinkling of sesame seeds, plus a pot of soy dressing to add when you're ready to eat.

● GH TIP
To make this dish gluten free, use tamari soy sauce.

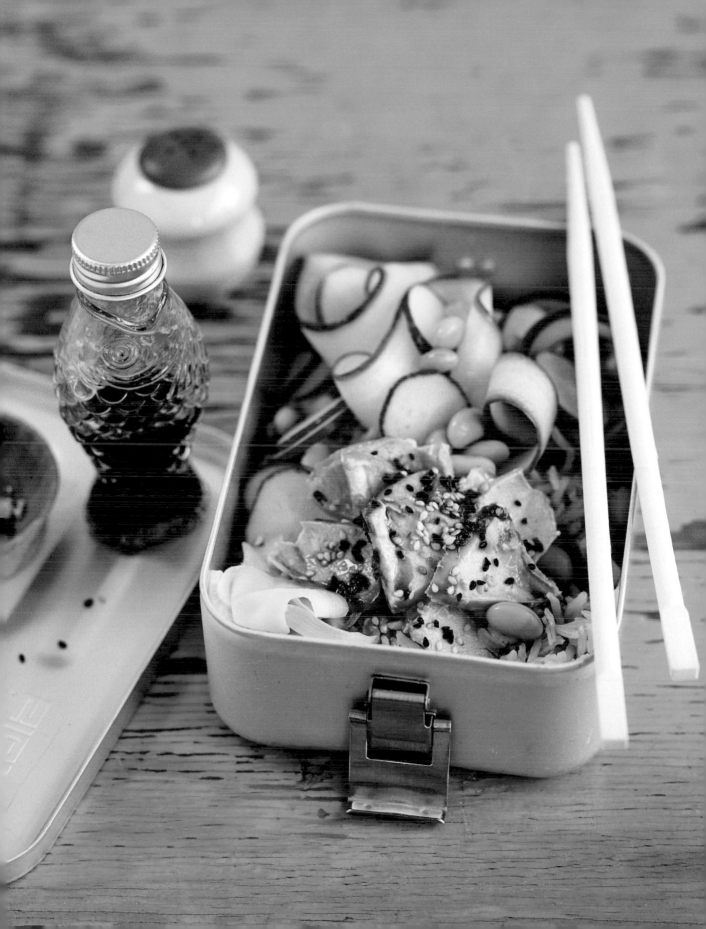

Prawn and Mango Noodle Salad

You only need to boil the kettle for this refreshing Vietnamese-style salad, making it an ideal supper for summer days when you'd rather not be stuck in the kitchen with a hot stove.

Hands-on time: 15 minutes
Serves 4

125g (4oz) dried rice vermicelli
    noodles
300g (11oz) cooked jumbo
    prawns
200g (7oz) sugar snap peas,
    halved
1 medium mango, peeled and
    chopped
Small bunch of fresh
    coriander, chopped
Small bunch of fresh mint,
    chopped
2 spring onions, finely sliced
25g (1oz) dry roasted peanuts,
    chopped

FOR THE DRESSING
2 tbsp sweet chilli sauce
Juice of 1 lime
1 tsp Thai fish sauce

**PER SERVING 280cals,
23g protein, 5g fat (1g
saturates), 34g carbs (8g
total sugars), 4g fibre**

1. Snap the noodles into quarters, then put into a large bowl and pour over freshly boiled water to cover. Set aside for 5 minutes, stirring to soften them. Drain the noodles into a sieve and rinse under running cold water to cool.

2. Meanwhile, mix together the dressing ingredients in a small bowl. Put the prawns into a large salad bowl or serving dish and toss with half the dressing. Add the noodles, sugar snap peas, mango and herbs to the bowl with the prawns and toss them together gently. Scatter over the spring onions and peanuts and serve with the remaining dressing alongside.

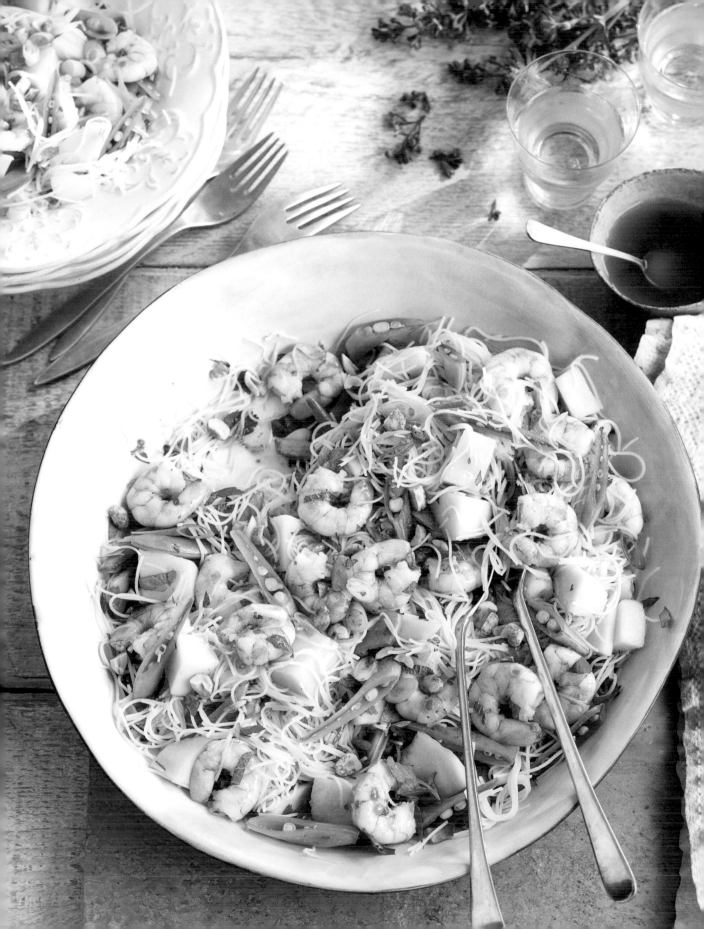

Asparagus, New Potato and Bacon Salad

This is a true celebration of spring – during April and May, seek out Jersey Royals and English asparagus for the best flavour.

Hands-on time: 20 minutes
Cooking time: about
   20 minutes
Serves 4

500g bag new potatoes, halved if large (use Jersey Royals, if available)
200g (7oz) frozen peas (or use fresh, if available)
250g (9oz) bunch British asparagus, ends trimmed
12 rashers smoked streaky bacon
75g bag pea shoots
75g (3oz) Lancashire cheese, crumbled

FOR THE SALSA VERDE
25g pack each fresh basil, parsley and fresh mint (stalks removed)
1 tbsp capers, drained and rinsed
3 anchovy fillets, from a tin
1 small garlic clove
1 tsp Dijon mustard
Juice of ½–1 lemon (to taste)
5 tbsp olive oil

PER SERVING 483cals, 22g protein, 31g fat (10g saturates), 26g carbs (6g total sugars), 7g fibre

1. Heat the grill to high. Bring a large pan of salted water to the boil, add the potatoes and cook for 15-20 minutes or until tender. Add the peas and asparagus for the final 5 minutes, then remove from the heat and drain well.

2. Meanwhile, grill the bacon for 2–3 minutes on each side until crispy, then transfer to kitchen paper to drain.

3. Make the dressing: in a small food processor, whiz the basil, parsley and mint leaves with the capers, anchovy fillets, garlic, mustard, lemon juice (to taste) and olive oil until combined but still chunky. Mix in 2–3 tablespoons cold water to thin, if needed. Season to taste.

4. Tip the potatoes and veg into a large bowl. Add half the dressing and half of the pea shoots, then season with freshly ground black pepper (the dressing will already be salty enough). Toss gently to combine.

5. Transfer the salad to a serving plate, top with the crispy bacon rashers and the remaining pea shoots, and crumble over the cheese. Serve with extra dressing on the side.

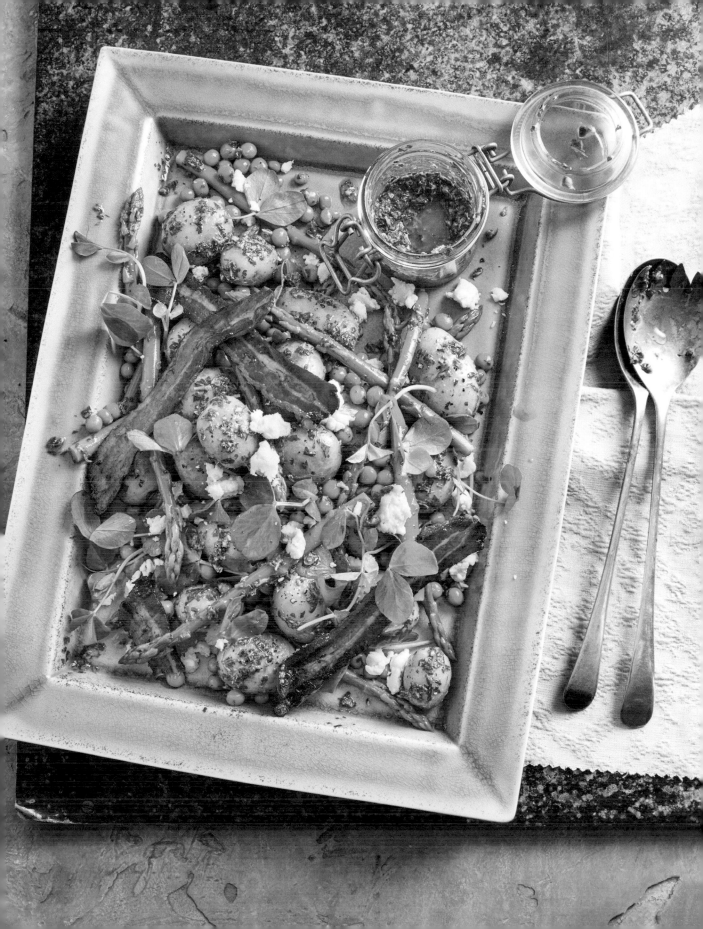

Kung Pao Turkey Wraps

These healthy wraps would work well with minced chicken or beef, too. Bring them to the table with the toppings on the side for your family or guests to assemble themselves.

Hands-on time: 10 minutes
Cooking time: about
   12 minutes
Serves 4

4 tbsp soy sauce
2 tbsp cornflour
2 tbsp sweet chilli sauce
3 tbsp mirin
2 tbsp sesame oil
500g (1lb 2oz) turkey mince
1 garlic clove, crushed
5cm (2in) piece fresh root
   ginger, finely grated
1 courgette, finely chopped
1 red pepper, finely sliced
Little Gem lettuce, leaves
   separated, to serve
3 spring onions, finely sliced,
   to serve
50g (2oz) salted peanuts,
   roughly chopped, to serve
Rice, to serve (optional)

PER SERVING 435cals,
41g protein, 21g fat (5g
saturates), 19g carbs (10g
total sugars), 3g fibre

1. In a small bowl, mix together 2 tablespoons of soy sauce, 1 tablespoon of cornflour, the sweet chilli sauce, mirin and 1 teaspoon of sesame oil with 1 tablespoon of water. Set aside.

2. Set a wok or large frying pan over medium heat. Add the remaining sesame oil to the pan with the turkey and the remaining soy sauce and cornflour. Stir-fry for 5 minutes until the turkey is dry and well coated.

3. Add the garlic, ginger, courgette and pepper to the pan and continue to fry for 5 minutes until the turkey is cooked through. Add the soy sauce mixture to the pan and stir to coat the turkey in the sauce – add up to 3 tablespoons of water if the mixture is too dry.

4. Serve the turkey in lettuce leaves with the spring onions, peanuts and rice, if you like, in separate bowls to be added to the wraps at the table.

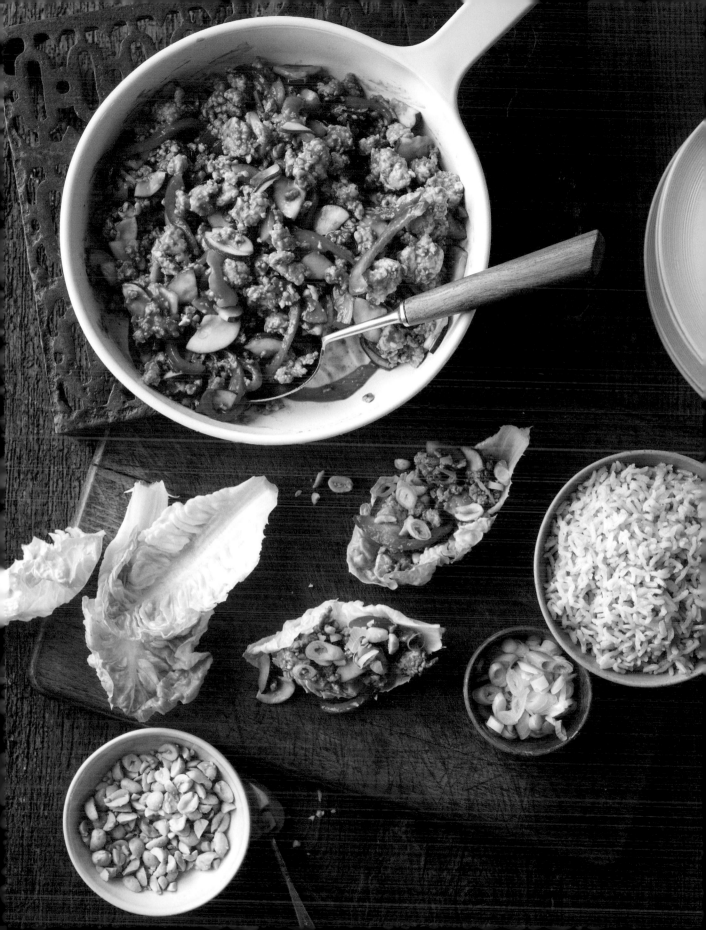

Lamb Fattoush

This hearty Middle Eastern salad includes toasted pitta breads. Marinating the lamb in a fragrant spice mix gives it a real flavour boost.

Hands-on time: 10 minutes
Cooking time: around
10 minutes
Serves 4

4 lamb leg steaks (about 450g/1lb), chopped into 2.5cm (1in) pieces
1 tbsp baharat or ras el hanout spice mix
4 tbsp olive oil
1 cucumber
½ small red onion, finely sliced
6 tomatoes, cut into wedges
200g (7oz) radishes, quartered
Bunch each fresh flat-leaf parsley and mint, roughly chopped
2 pitta breads, toasted and roughly chopped
1 small garlic clove, crushed
Juice of ½ lemon

PER SERVING 402cals, 28g protein, 21g fat (6g saturates), 23g carbs (8g total sugars), 4g fibre

1. If using wooden skewers, soak them in cold water for a few minutes to stop them from burning under the grill. In a bowl, mix the lamb with the spice mix, 1 tablespoon of the oil and some seasoning. Set aside to marinate while you prepare the salad.

2. Halve and deseed the cucumber, then slice it into half-moons. Put into a large bowl or serving dish with the onion, tomatoes, radishes, herbs and toasted pitta. For the dressing, whisk together the remaining olive oil with the garlic, lemon juice and some seasoning. Pour over the salad and toss together.

3. Heat the grill to medium-high. Take the lamb chunks out of the marinade and thread them on to metal or the pre-soaked wooden skewers. Grill the skewers for 8–10 minutes, turning occasionally, until cooked to your liking. Serve the skewers with the salad.

● GH TIP
Make it veggie: swap the lamb for vegetables such as red peppers, courgettes and aubergines, with or without halloumi.

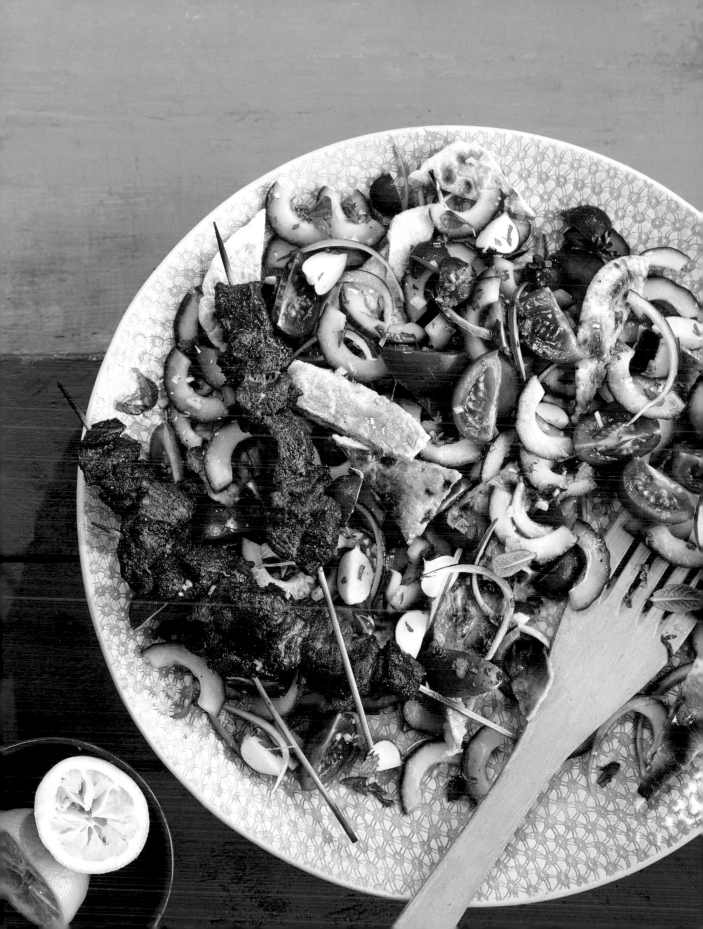

Chicken Shawarma Flatbreads

Aromatic, peppery baharat (a spice blend that includes paprika, coriander, cinnamon and cardamom) brings masses of flavour to this dish without the need for lots of ingredients – find it in the spice aisle at larger supermarkets.

Hands-on time: 15 minutes
Cooking time: about
   10 minutes
Serves 4

600g (1lb 5oz) skinless, boneless chicken thighs
Large handful of fresh coriander
1 tbsp baharat spice mix
Finely grated zest and juice of 1 lemon
1 tbsp olive oil
4 small wholemeal flatbreads, to serve
100g hummus, to serve

FOR THE SLAW
½ small red cabbage, thinly sliced
1 small red onion, thinly sliced
¼ cucumber, deseeded and sliced

PER SERVING 476cals, 33g protein, 26g fat (5g saturates), 26g carbs (5g total sugars), 4g fibre

1. Trim any excess fat from the chicken thighs and set one on a board sandwiched between 2 sheets of clingfilm. Lightly bash it with a rolling pin until 1cm (½in) thick. Repeat with the remaining chicken, then transfer the flattened thighs to a non-metallic bowl. On a clean board, finely chop the coriander stalks and leaves, keeping them separate. Add the stalks to the bowl with the chicken, followed by the baharat, lemon zest and olive oil. Toss to coat the chicken well and set aside.

2. Tip the cabbage, onion, cucumber and most of the chopped coriander leaves into a bowl. Toss with the lemon juice and set aside

3. Heat the grill to medium. Spread out the chicken thighs on a wire rack set over a baking sheet and grill for 3–5 minutes on each side, brushing them with any excess marinade, until cooked through. Transfer to a chopping board and finely slice the meat.

4. To serve, spread each flatbread with a layer of hummus, top with some slaw and chicken, then sprinkle over the remaining coriander leaves.

◆ GET AHEAD
Make the slaw up to 3 hours in advance and store in a non-metallic bowl. Marinate the chicken (step 1) up to a day beforehand, then store in a non-metallic bowl, covered, in the fridge. Bring to room temperature before completing the recipe to serve.

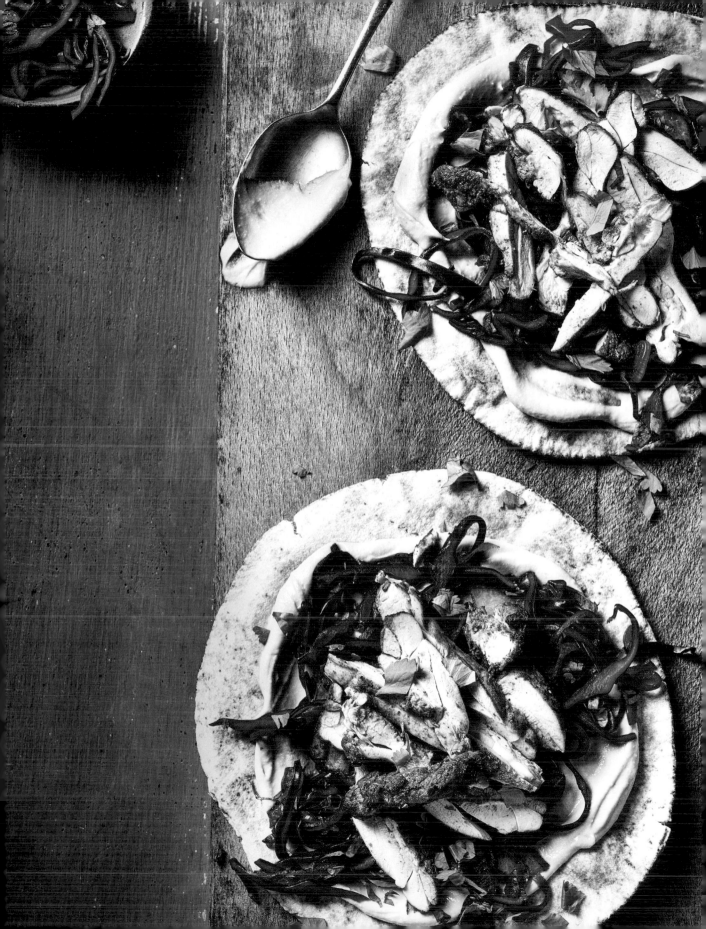

Skinny Hawaiian Pizzas

Enjoy a midweek lower-carb pizza by using tortilla wraps rather than the traditional base. Preheat the baking trays to get the tortillas nice and crispy.

Hands-on time: 10 minutes
Cooking time: about
   7 minutes
Serves 4

4 flour tortilla wraps
175ml (6fl oz) onion and garlic
   passata
125g (4oz) wafer-thin ham
227g tin pineapple slices,
   drained and cut into chunks
70g bag rocket
125g (4oz) ball light
   mozzarella, roughly torn
4 tsp balsamic glaze, to drizzle
Salad leaves, to serve
   (optional)

PER SERVING 221cals,
13g protein, 5g fat (3g
saturates), 31g carbs (6g
total sugars), 2g fibre

1. Put two large, rimless baking trays in the oven and preheat to 220°C (200°C fan) mark 7.

2. Cut 2 pieces of baking parchment, each larger than the baking trays. Put 2 tortillas alongside each other on each piece. Spread each tortilla with 2 tablespoons passata, leaving a 1cm (½in) gap around the edges. Evenly scatter over the ham and pineapple, then season well.

3. Carefully transfer the tortillas to the baking trays and cook for 5–7 minutes until the bases are crispy and golden. To serve, top each tortilla pizza with a handful of rocket and mozzarella, then drizzle over 1 teaspoon balsamic glaze. Serve with salad leaves, if you like.

Chicken Naan Salad

Classic curry flavours transform this chicken salad, and it's a great choice for lunchboxes or a light supper.

Hands-on time: 10 minutes
Cooking time: about
   10 minutes
Serves 4

4 skinless, boneless chicken
   breasts
3 tbsp mild curry paste
Large bunch of fresh
   coriander, stalks and leaves
50g (2oz) natural yogurt
2 tbsp mango chutney
Juice of ½ lime
3 large carrots
1 cucumber
3 tomatoes
2 naan breads

PER SERVING 452cals, 39g
protein, 9g fat (1g
saturates), 50g carbs (15g
total sugars), 6g fibre

1. Put the chicken breasts between 2 sheets of baking paper and bash with a rolling pin to an even thickness of 1cm (½in). Rub the curry paste over the meat.

2. Set a large griddle or frying pan over medium-high heat and cook the chicken for about 5 minutes on each side or until cooked through.

3. Meanwhile, in the small bowl of a food processor or blender, whiz most of the coriander leaves (set aside a few to use as a garnish) and the stalks with the yogurt, chutney, lime juice and some seasoning. Set aside.

4. Heat the grill. Working over a large serving platter, peel the carrots and cucumber into long ribbons using a Y-shaped vegetable peeler (stop when you reach the cucumber seeds, which can be discarded). Chop the tomatoes into wedges and dot over the salad.

5. Grill the naans according to the pack instructions. Slice the naans and chicken into strips and add to the salad platter. Drizzle over the coriander yogurt dressing and sprinkle with the remaining coriander leaves to serve.

Sweet-and-sour Chicken

Tinned pineapple adds a fruity hit to this Friday-night favourite.

Hands-on time: 10 minutes
Cooking time: around
   10 minutes
Serves 4

250g (9oz) dry medium egg
   noodles
1 tbsp vegetable oil
400g (14oz) skinless chicken
   breast, diced
5cm (2in) piece fresh root
   ginger, grated
300g pack mixed stir-fry
   vegetables of your choice,
   chopped if large
1½ tbsp cornflour
5 tbsp sweet chilli sauce
½ tbsp soy sauce
2 tbsp white wine vinegar
227g tin pineapple rings,
   roughly chopped, with
   3 tbsp juice reserved
Large handful of beansprouts
Large handful of fresh
   coriander, leaves picked

PER SERVING 483cals,
36g protein, 9g fat (2g
saturates), 63g carbs (14g
total sugars), 3g fibre

1. Bring a pan of water to the boil and cook the noodles according to the pack instructions. Drain, then tip back into the pan to keep warm.

2. Meanwhile, put the oil in a wok or large frying pan set over high heat. Add the chicken and stir-fry for 5 minutes until golden. Stir in the ginger, mixed vegetables and a splash of water. Continue to stir-fry until the vegetables are just tender and the chicken is cooked through.

3. Put the cornflour into a small bowl and gradually whisk in the sweet chilli and soy sauces, then the vinegar and reserved pineapple juice until smooth. Add the cornflour mixture and pineapple chunks to the chicken pan and cook, stirring occasionally, until the sauce is thick and syrupy, about 30 seconds.

4. Check the seasoning and sprinkle over the beansprouts and coriander leaves. Serve immediately with the noodles.

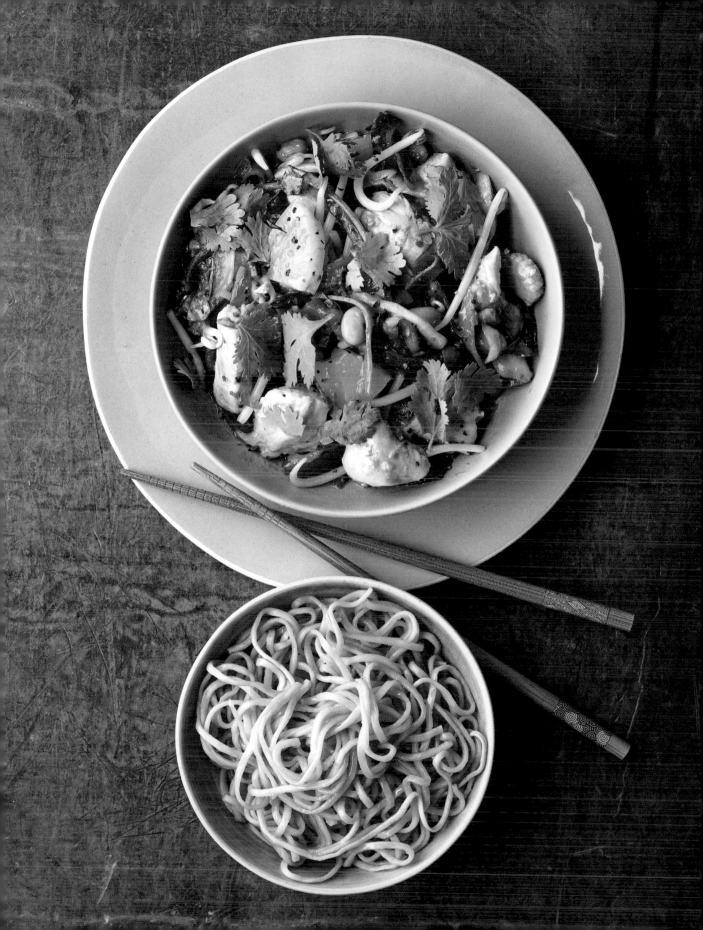

Pork Fried Rice

Use chicken or prawns in place of the pork shoulder in this versatile dish.

Hands-on time: 15 minutes
Cooking time: about
**   15 minutes**
Serves 4

3 eggs, beaten gently
1 tbsp sesame oil
500g (1lb 2oz) diced pork
    shoulder
1 large carrot, peeled and
    finely chopped
1 garlic clove, crushed
150g (5oz) peas
100g (3½oz) tinned sweetcorn,
    drained
2 x 250g pouches ready-
    cooked rice
1½ tbsp soy sauce
1 tsp Thai fish sauce
2 tbsp sweet chilli sauce
2 spring onions, finely sliced
Large handful of fresh
    coriander, roughly chopped

PER SERVING 445cals,
31g protein, 28g fat (8g
saturates), 15g carbs (8g
total sugars), 5g fibre

1. Set a large non-stick frying pan or wok over a low heat and cook the eggs, stirring frequently, until scrambled and just cooked through. Transfer to a plate.

2. Heat the oil in the pan, add the pork and fry for 5 minutes until golden. Add the carrot and cook for 5 minutes until it and the meat are cooked through. Add the garlic and cook for a further minute.

3. Stir through the peas, sweetcorn, rice, soy and fish sauces, sweet chilli, most of the spring onions and most of the coriander along with the scrambled eggs. Serve immediately, garnished with the remaining spring onions and coriander.

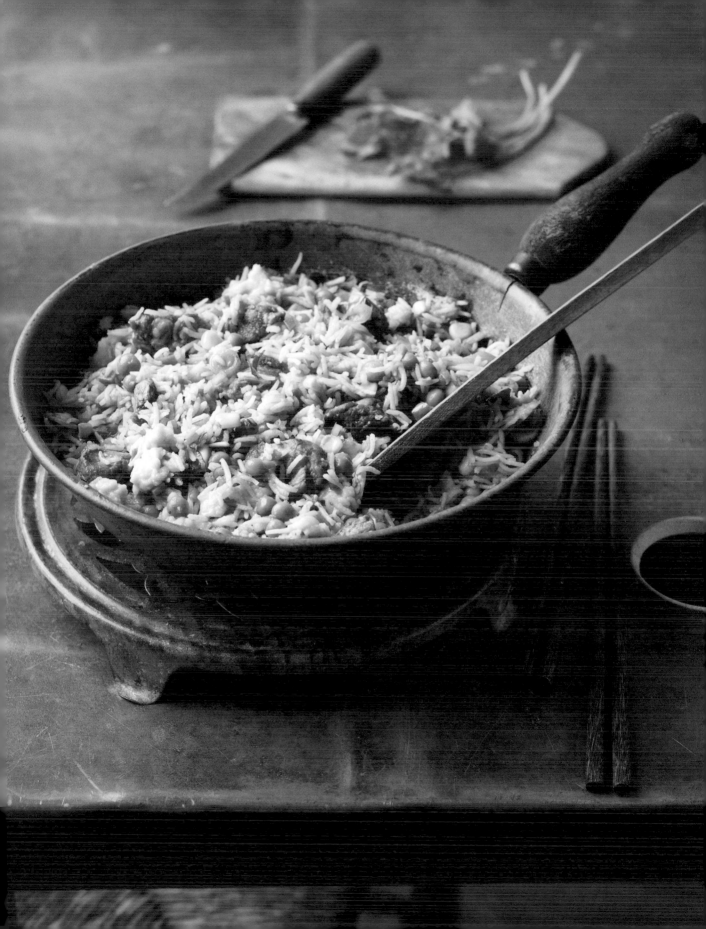

Korean Steak Slaw

Gochujang, a Korean chilli paste, adds a sweet and spicy kick to this salad. It's available in most large supermarkets, but if you can't find it, sriracha hot sauce makes a good substitute. You can also use it to spice up your greens — see page 164.

Hands-on time: 15 minutes
Cooking time: about
**   5 minutes**
Serves 4

2 tbsp gochujang Korean
    spice paste or sriracha hot
    sauce
2 tbsp soy sauce
3 tbsp sesame oil
2 sirloin steaks, trimmed of
    fat, about 450g (1lb)
1 mooli (see GH Tip)
1 large carrot
½ red cabbage
5 spring onions
2 tbsp rice vinegar
2 tsp toasted sesame seeds

PER SERVING 301cals,
29g protein, 15g fat (4g
saturates), 11g carbs (10g
total sugars), 3g fibre

1. In a large bowl, mix together the gochujang or sriracha, soy sauce and 2 tablespoons of sesame oil to make a marinade. Put 1 tablespoon of the marinade in a jug and set aside to use in the dressing, then add the steaks to the bowl and mix well to coat in the remaining marinade. Set aside for a few minutes to soak.

2. Meanwhile, use a julienne peeler to peel the mooli and carrot into strips. Shred the red cabbage very finely (use a mandoline if you have one) and finely slice 3 of the spring onions into strips. Put all of the vegetables into a large bowl. Mix the reserved marinade with the remaining sesame oil and the rice vinegar to make a dressing, then pour over the vegetable slaw and toss to coat.

3. Heat a griddle or frying pan until very hot. Remove the steaks from the marinade (reserve the marinade) and fry them for 2 minutes on each side for medium rare, brushing them with the reserved marinade as they cook. If you prefer your steak well done, fry for a further minute on each side. Set the steaks aside to rest on a board for 5 minutes, then slice into thin strips. Meanwhile, finely slice the remaining spring onions and add these to the slaw.

4. Serve the slaw with the sliced steak on the side, sprinkled with the toasted sesame seeds.

● GH TIP
Mooli, or daikon, is a large white radish. If it's not available, finely slice half a white or Chinese cabbage instead.

◆ GET AHEAD
Marinate the steak for up to 2 hours before cooking.

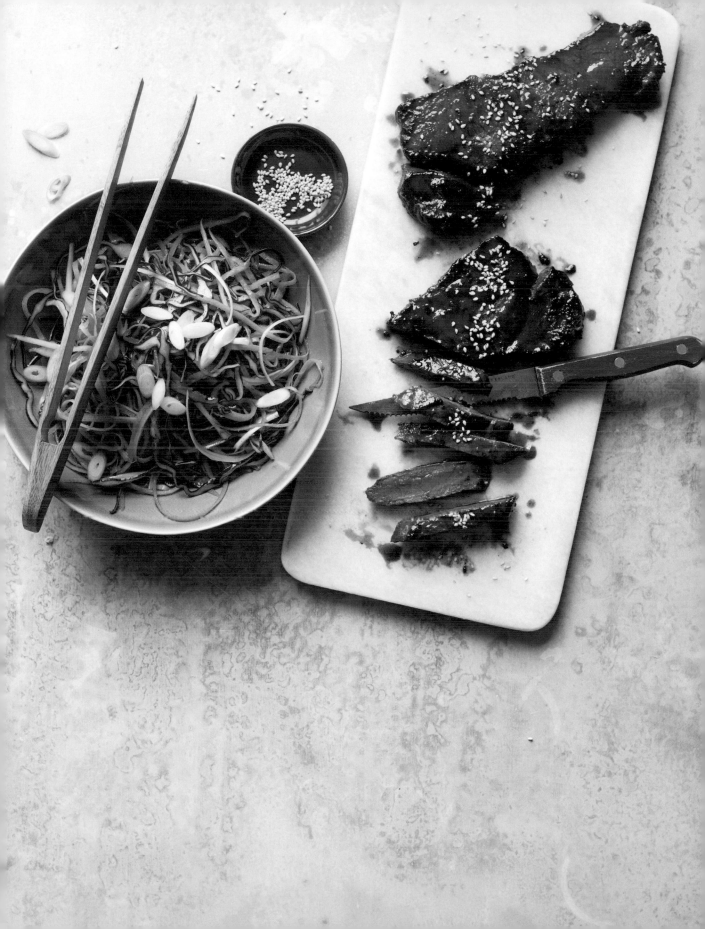

Butterbean and Prawn Saganaki

Our speedy version of this Greek dish includes filling butterbeans to boost your five-a-day. If you're not making it gluten free, serve it with crusty bread to soak up the delicious sauce.

Hands-on time: 5 minutes
Cooking time: about
   15 minutes
Serves 4

1 tbsp olive oil
1 onion, finely chopped
2 garlic cloves, crushed
125ml (4fl oz) white wine
400g tin chopped tomatoes
400g tin butter beans, drained
   and rinsed
Pinch of dried chilli flakes
Pinch of sugar
300g (11oz) raw king pawns
100g (3½oz) feta cheese
Small bunch of fresh dill,
   chopped
Crusty bread, to serve
   (optional; see introduction)

PER SERVING 261cals,
22g protein, 9g fat (4g
saturates), 15g carbs (7g
total sugars), 6g fibre

1. Put the oil in an ovenproof frying pan set over medium heat. Fry the onion for 5 minutes until softened. Add the garlic and cook for a further minute. Increase the heat, then add the wine, tomatoes and beans with a pinch of chilli flakes and sugar. Season well. Bring to the boil and bubble for 5 minutes to reduce slightly.

2. Heat the grill to high. Stir the prawns into the sauce, crumble over the feta, then set the pan under the grill for about 5 minutes until the prawns are pink and cheese begins to turn golden. Sprinkle with dill and serve with crusty bread, if you like.

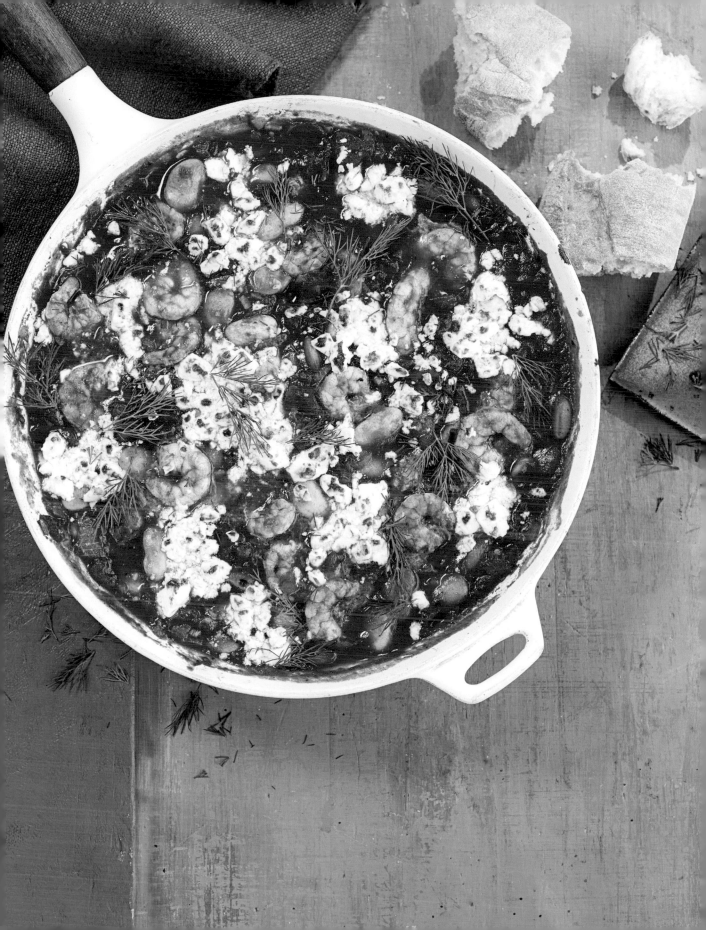

Sicilian All-in-One Pasta

The starch released while the pasta cooks mixes with the other ingredients to make a velvety sauce.

Hands-on time: 10 minutes
Cooking time: about
15 minutes
Serves 4

300g (11oz) wholewheat
   spaghetti
400g (14oz) cherry tomatoes
Finely grated zest and juice of
   1 orange
50ml (2fl oz) olive oil
50g (2oz) sultanas
5cm (2in) cinnamon stick
2 fresh oregano sprigs, leaves
   picked, plus extra to garnish
160g tin tuna in spring water,
   drained
Large handful of rocket

PER SERVING 449cals,
22g protein, 12g fat (2g
saturates), 60g carbs (15g
total sugars), 10g fibre

1. Put the spaghetti into a large, deep frying pan so it lies flat – breaking it up, if necessary. Add the tomatoes, orange zest and juice, oil, sultanas, cinnamon, oregano and some seasoning.

2. Pour over 750ml (1¼ pints) freshly boiled water from the kettle. Bring up to the boil over high heat, then bubble for about 15 minutes, stirring occasionally, or until the pasta is just tender and there is a nice volume of sauce left.

3. Mix through the tuna and check the seasoning. Discard the cinnamon stick. Divide the spaghetti among 4 bowls and sprinkle over some oregano leaves and rocket. Serve.

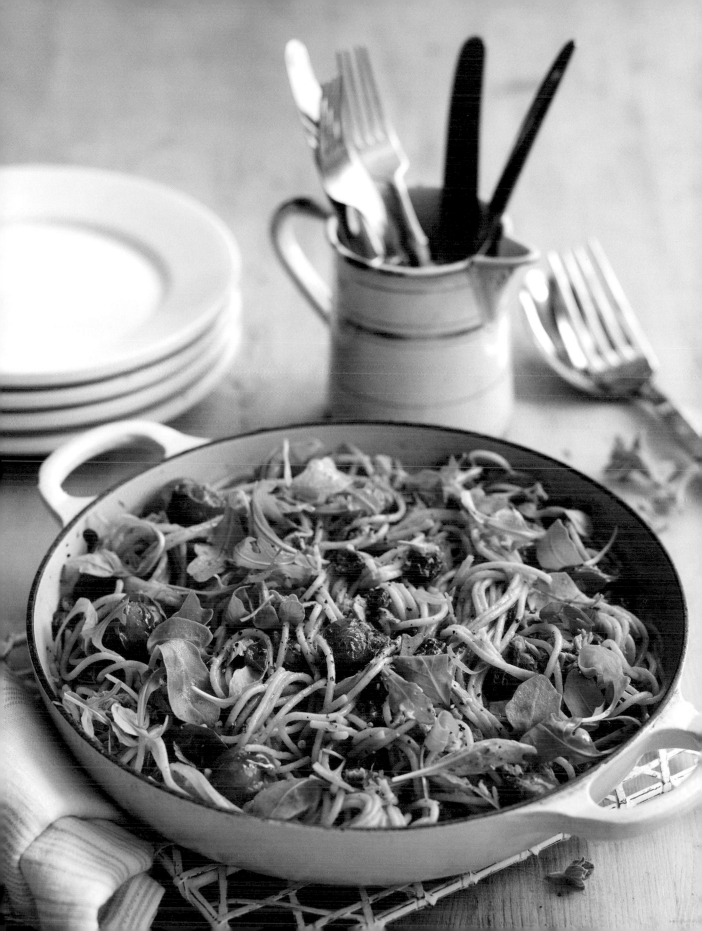

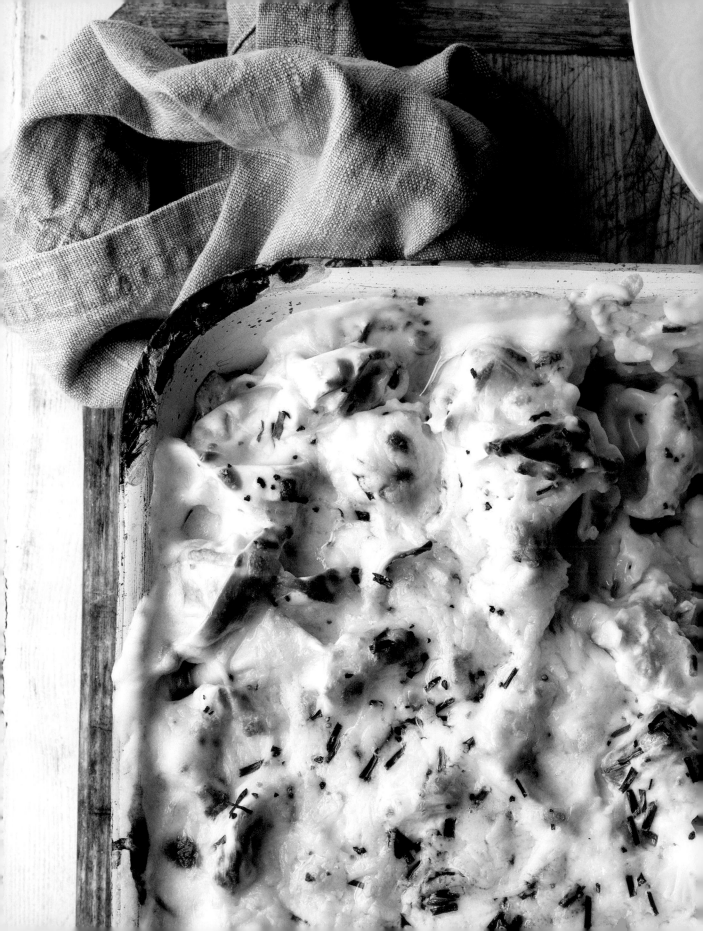

Quick Comfort

Grilled Swiss Cheese and Ham Hock Sandwich

This glamorous version of the classic cheese toastie is a real treat when you're in need of something warming and satisfying.

Hands-on time: 5 minutes
Cooking time: 10 minutes
Makes 2 sandwiches

2 tsp soft butter
4 slices sourdough bread
2 tbsp wholegrain mustard
4 gherkins, sliced
200g (7oz) ham hock,
　shredded
200g (7oz) Gruyère cheese,
　grated

PER SERVING 556cals,
33g protein, 30g fat (17g
saturates), 39g carbs (2g
total sugars), 4g fibre

1. Set a frying pan over medium heat. Spread the butter on one side of all 4 bread slices, then turn the slices over and spread each with mustard. Layer 2 of the bread slices with sliced gherkins, shredded ham hock and grated cheese, then sandwich together with the remaining bread slices, butter side out.

2. Cook the sandwiches in the pan for 4–5 minutes on each side, pressing or weighting them down until the bread is toasted and the filling is melted and hot throughout.

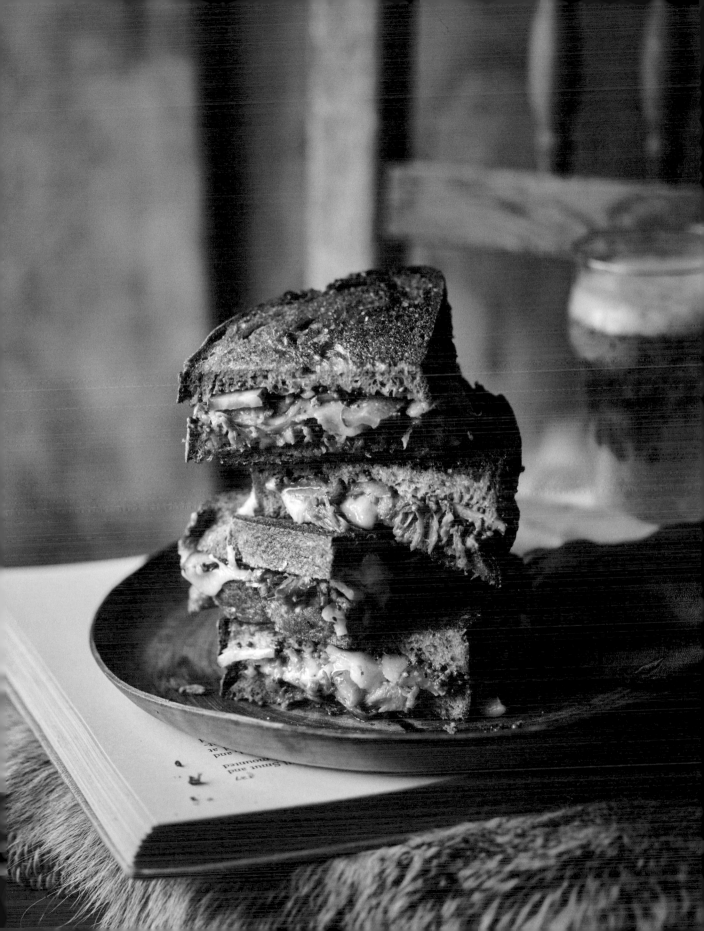

Shrimp Po'boy

A po'boy is a traditional sandwich from Louisiana that most often includes deep-fried meat or seafood served up in a crusty French loaf. We've chosen king prawns (or 'shrimp') for our taste of the deep south.

Hands-on time: 20 minutes
Cooking time: about
   10 minutes
Serves 2

100g (3½oz) plain flour
1 tsp garlic granules
½ tsp cayenne pepper
150ml (¼ pint) buttermilk (or see GH tip)
150g (5oz) raw peeled king prawns
Vegetable oil, to fry
25g (1oz) each red and white cabbage, shredded
2 tbsp mayonnaise
2 tsp hot sauce, plus extra to drizzle (optional)
2 submarine rolls
Little Gem lettuce leaves, to serve

PER SERVING 673cals, 25g protein, 26g fat (3g saturates), 83g carbs (7g total sugars), 5g fibre

1. In a large bowl, mix the flour, garlic granules and cayenne pepper with 1 teaspoon salt. Measure the buttermilk into a small bowl. Pat the prawns dry with kitchen paper. Working a few at a time, dip the prawns into the buttermilk, then toss in the flour mixture.

2. Fill a heavy-based pan one-third full with oil and heat to 180°C, as measured on a cooking thermometer, or until a cube of bread sizzles to golden in 40 seconds. Fry the coated prawns for 4 minutes, turning occasionally, until crispy and golden. Lift out with a slotted spoon on to kitchen paper to drain.

3. Mix the shredded cabbages with the mayonnaise, hot sauce and some seasoning. Slice down into the top of each submarine roll. Fill the gap with a few lettuce leaves, half the cabbage mixture and prawns. Drizzle with extra hot sauce, if you like, and serve.

● GH TIP
If you don't have buttermilk, add 1 teaspoon of lemon juice to a measuring cup and top up with milk to make 150ml (¼ pint). Set aside for 5 minutes, then use in place of buttermilk in the recipe.

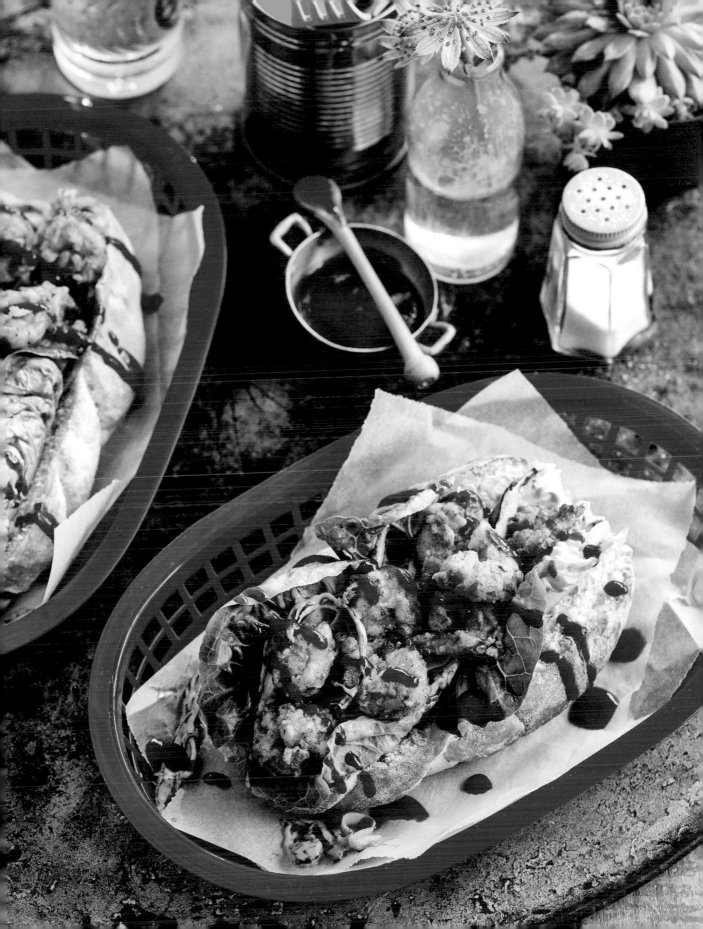

Tuna-melt Nachos

As the tortilla chips at the bottom of this dish will soften during baking, think of this melt as a Mexican-style lasagne.

GF

Hands-on time: 15 minutes
Cooking time: about
15 minutes
Serves 4

1 tbsp sunflower oil
1 red onion, finely chopped
1 garlic clove, crushed
2 green chillies, 1 finely
   chopped and 1 sliced
400g tin chopped tomatoes
½ tsp caster sugar
2 x 160g tins tuna in spring
   water, drained
Small bunch of fresh
   coriander, roughly chopped
200g (7oz) plain tortilla chips
125g (4oz) strong Cheddar,
   coarsely grated
75g (3oz) ready-made
   guacamole
2 spring onions, sliced

PER SERVING 516cals,
28g protein, 28g fat (10g
saturates), 36g carbs (6g
total sugars), 6g fibre

1. Preheat the oven to 220°C (200°C fan) mark 7. Put the oil in a large frying pan set over medium heat, then fry the onion for 5 minutes. Add the garlic and finely chopped chilli and fry for 1 minute. Stir in the tomatoes, sugar, tuna and most of the coriander. Check the seasoning.

2. Arrange half the tortilla chips in the base of a deep ovenproof dish. Top with half the tuna mixture and scatter over half the cheese. Repeat with another layer of the remaining tortillas, tuna mixture and cheese.

3. Cook in the oven for 10 minutes until piping hot and the cheese has melted. Dot the surface with dollops of guacamole and scatter over the sliced chilli, spring onions and remaining coriander. Serve immediately.

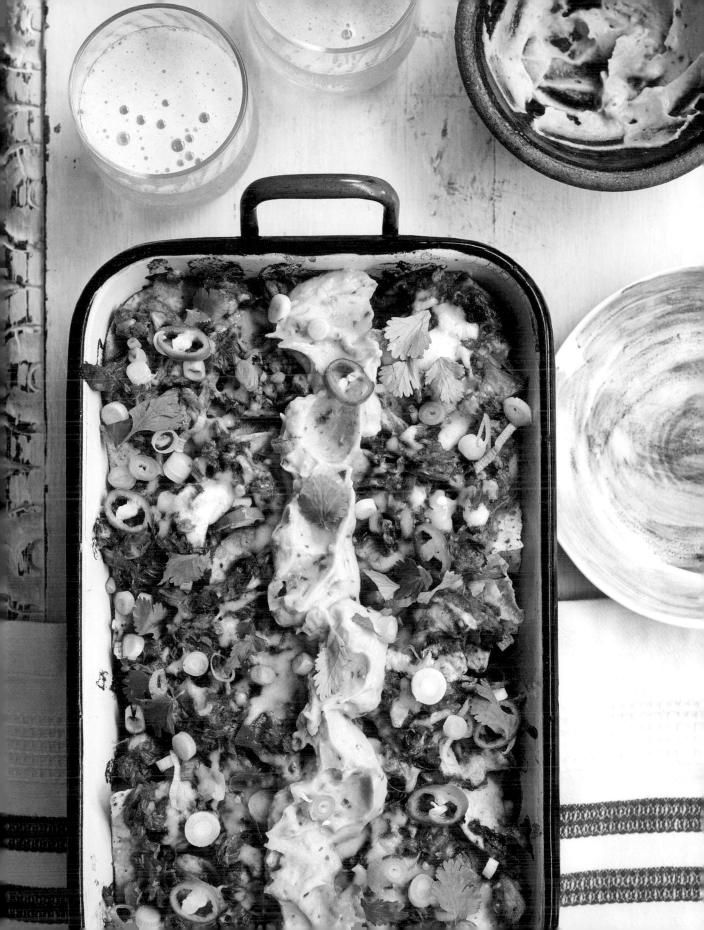

Gammon and Cauliflower Cheese Grills

This recipe uses cream cheese to make a rich sauce that saves on prep time.

Hands-on time: 10 minutes
Cooking time: 15 minutes
Serves 4

4 x 250g (9oz) smoked
    gammon steaks
1 tsp sunflower oil
450g (1lb) cauliflower florets
    (halved if large)
75g (3oz) mature Cheddar
    cheese, finely grated
200g (7oz) cream cheese
1 tsp gluten-free English
    mustard
1 medium egg
Few dashes of Worcestershire
    sauce
1 tbsp chopped fresh chives,
    plus extra to garnish

PER SERVING 711cals,
56g protein, 52g fat (26g
saturates), 3g carbs (3g total
sugars), 3g fibre

1. Heat the grill to high. Line a large baking tray with foil. Snip any fat on the edge of each gammon steak at 2cm (¼in) intervals, then brush the steaks with oil. Put on a lined baking tray and grill for 8–10 minutes or until cooked through, turning halfway through the cooking time.

2. Meanwhile, bring a pan of lightly salted water up to the boil. Add the cauliflower and simmer for 4–5 minutes until tender. Drain and leave to steam dry while you make the sauce.

3. In a large bowl, stir together the remaining ingredients, then add the cauliflower and stir until combined. Spoon a quarter of the mixture on top of each gammon steak. Grill for a further 5 minutes until golden and bubbling. Scatter over a few more chives and serve with a green salad.

● GH TIP
Some brands of prepared sauces may include gluten as a thickener – be sure to check the labels if you are cooking for those on a special diet.

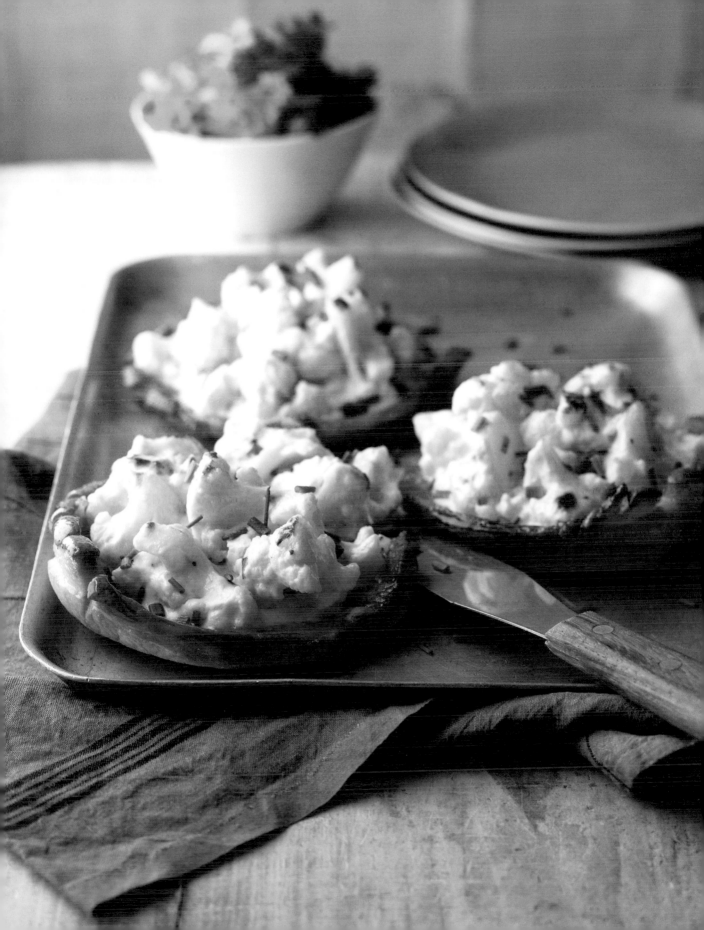

Chicken and Bacon Turnovers

A great way to use up leftover cooked chicken. These turnovers need just a quick assembly job, so will be on the table in 30 minutes!

Hands-on time: 10 minutes
Cooking time: 20 minutes
Serves 4

180g tub cream cheese
1 tsp English mustard
3 skinless cooked chicken
  breasts, finely chopped
25g (1oz) cooked crispy bacon,
  chopped
2 tbsp chopped fresh chives
75g (3oz) sweetcorn (either
  tinned or frozen, defrosted
  if frozen)
320g ready-rolled puff pastry
  sheet
1 medium egg, beaten

PER SERVING 682cals,
**37g protein, 49g fat (26g
saturates), 24g carbs (1g
total sugars), 2g fibre**

1. Preheat the oven to 220°C (200°C fan) mark 7. In a large bowl, beat the cream cheese until soft. Stir in the mustard, chicken, bacon, chives and sweetcorn and season to taste.

2. Unroll the pastry sheet and use a rolling pin to flatten it a bit further to a rectangle about 28 x 38cm (11 x 15in). Cut the sheet into 4 quarters. Spoon a quarter of the filling on to one side of each pastry rectangle, leaving a 1cm (½in) border of pastry around the filling. Brush the pastry around the filling with beaten egg, then fold the other side of the pastry over the filling to cover it. Press the pastry together with your fingers to seal it, then use the tines of a fork to crimp the edges. Brush the top of the turnover with more egg and cut a steam hole in the centre. Repeat with the remaining pastry rectangles and filling to make 4 turnovers.

3. Arrange the turnovers on a baking sheet lined with baking paper, and cook for 20 minutes until puffed and golden. Leave to cool for a few minutes, then serve with a green salad.

● GH TIP
After brushing the tops of the turnovers with beaten egg, sprinkle over a few sesame or poppy seeds before cooking.

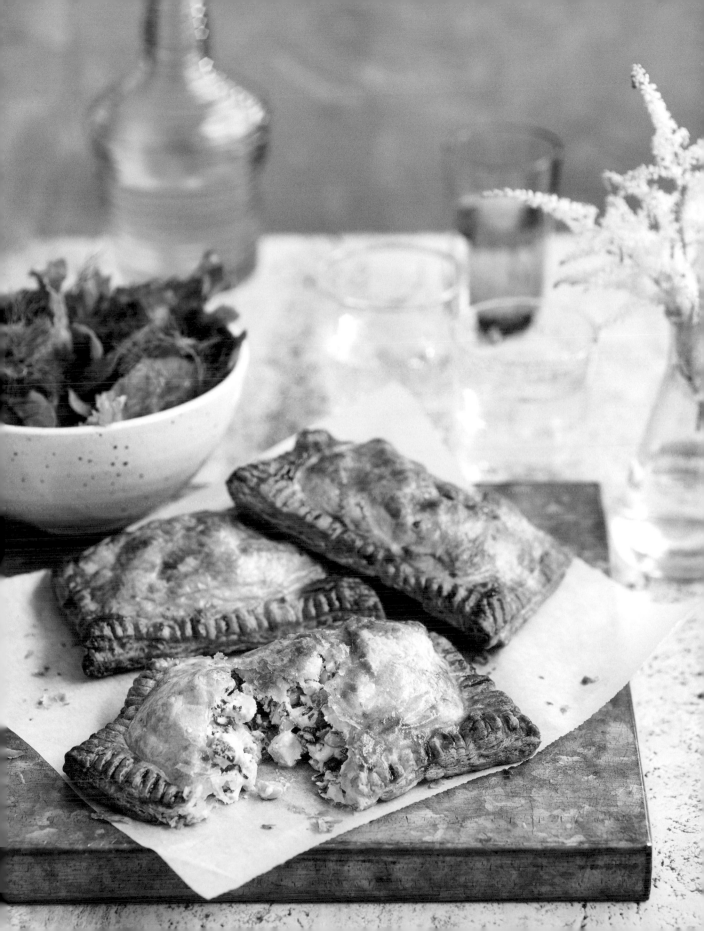

Bibimbap

This vibrant Korean rice dish is a wonderful way to use up leftovers — include any cooked vegetables, rice or meat you may have in the fridge in place of the fresh ingredients.

Hands-on time: 10 minutes
Cooking time: 20 minutes
Serves 4

300g (11oz) white rice
500g (1lb 2oz) beef mince
2 tbsp soy sauce
3 tbsp white wine vinegar
1 tbsp light brown sugar
2 garlic cloves, crushed
2 tbsp toasted sesame oil
2 carrots, finely sliced
2 courgettes, finely sliced
150g (5oz) bean sprouts
100g (3½oz) shiitake
   mushrooms, roughly sliced
125g (4oz) spinach
2 tbsp vegetable oil
4 eggs
Sesame seeds, to serve

FOR THE SAUCE
1 tbsp toasted sesame oil
1 tbsp light brown sugar
2 tsp white wine vinegar
2 tbsp gochujang Korean
   spice paste or sweet
   chilli sauce

PER SERVING 738cals,
34g protein, 30g fat (10g
saturates), 81g carbs (15g
total sugars), 4g fibre

1. In a medium pan, cook the white rice according to the pack instructions. Meanwhile, mix together the mince, soy sauce, white wine vinegar, brown sugar, crushed garlic and plenty of seasoning. Set aside.

2. In a large frying pan, heat 1 tablespoon sesame oil and fry the sliced carrots and courgettes for 5–6 minutes until just tender. Remove to a large plate near the hob. Add a further 1 tablespoon of sesame oil to the pan and fry the bean sprouts and shiitake mushrooms for 2–3 minutes, then transfer to the vegetable plate. Into the empty pan, add the beef mixture with any liquid and fry for 5–8 minutes until browned and cooked through. Add the spinach to the pan in batches, stirring to wilt. Remove the pan from the heat and keep warm.

3. Meanwhile, in a separate frying pan, heat the vegetable oil, crack in the eggs and fry to your liking.

4. Mix all the sauce ingredients together in a small bowl. To serve, divide the rice among 4 bowls and top each portion with the beef mixture, vegetables and a fried egg. Sprinkle over sesame seeds.

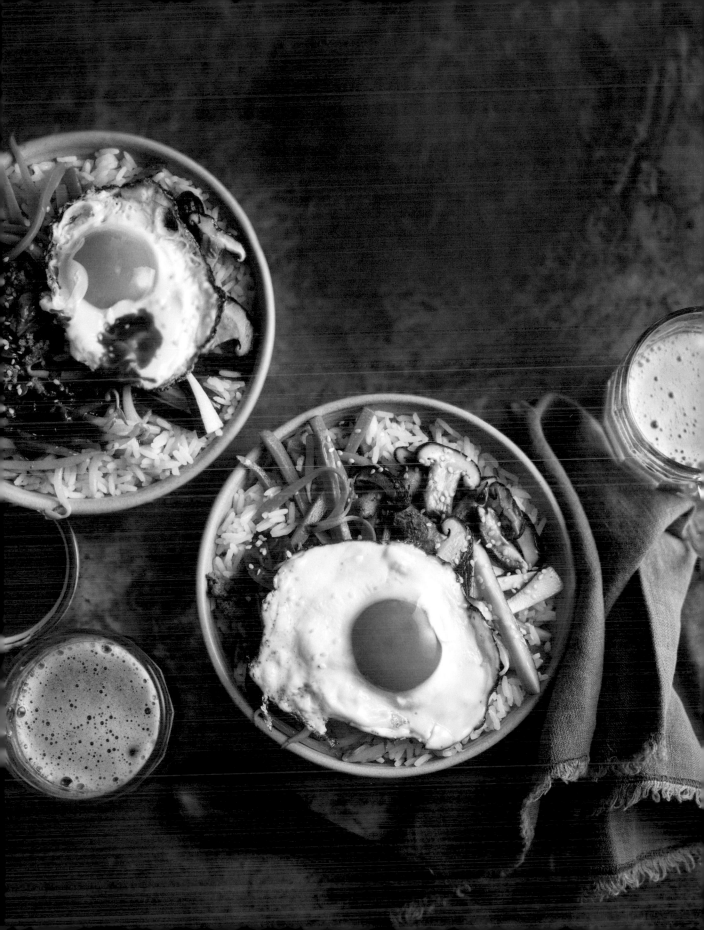

Smoked Salmon Gnocchi

This luxurious sauce and the fresh flavours of salmon and watercress would be delicious with any type of cooked pasta.

Hands-on time: 10 minutes
Cooking time: about
   10 minutes
Serves 6

1kg (2lb 2oz) gnocchi
300g (11oz) medium-fat cream
   cheese with herbs
1 large courgette, chopped
Finely grated zest of 1 lemon
125g (4oz) smoked salmon,
   chopped
Large handful of watercress

PER SERVING 403cals,
25g protein, 10g fat (4g
saturates), 53g carbs (3g
total sugars), 3g fibre

1. Cook the gnocchi in a large pan of boiling water according to the pack instructions (or until the gnocchi bob to the surface). Drain well, reserving a little of the cooking water.

2. In the empty gnocchi pan, heat the cream cheese, courgette and lemon zest until piping hot. Tip the gnocchi back into the pan and stir to coat in the sauce, adding a little of the reserved cooking water to loosen, if needed. Stir in the smoked salmon, most of the watercress and plenty of freshly ground black pepper. Check the seasoning and serve immediately, topped with a little more watercress.

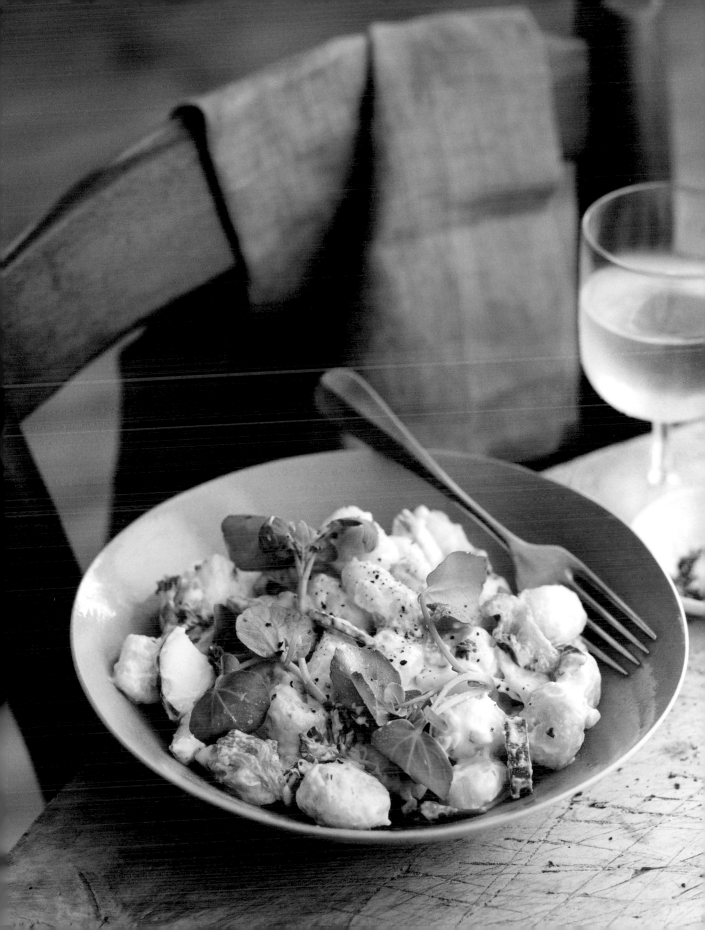

Weeknight Chicken Parmigiana

Bashing the chicken with a rolling pin tenderises the meat and helps it to cook more quickly. Serve this classic with a simple salad, or have it with pasta for a heartier dinner.

Hands-on time: 10 minutes
Cooking time: 20 minutes
Serves 4

700g (1½lb) tomato and basil
　　sauce
400g tin chopped tomatoes
4 chicken breasts
50g (2oz) plain flour
75g (3oz) breadcrumbs
50g (2oz) finely grated
　　Parmesan
2 medium eggs
3 tbsp olive oil
1 x 125g (4oz) ball mozzarella,
　　drained and thinly sliced
Fresh basil leaves, to serve

PER SERVING 623cals,
48g protein, 30g fat (10g
saturates), 38g carbs (15g
total sugars), 5g fibre

1. Pour the tomato sauce and chopped tomatoes into a pan and set over a low heat while you prepare the chicken.

2. Put the chicken breasts on a board and cover them with clingfilm, then bash them with a rolling pin until 1cm (½in) thick. Put the flour and some seasoning into a shallow bowl. In another bowl, mix the breadcrumbs with the Parmesan. In a third bowl, lightly beat the eggs. Coat each chicken breast in flour, tap off the excess, then dip it into the egg before coating it in breadcrumb mixture.

3. Heat the oil in a large frying pan and fry the chicken for 3 minutes on each side, or until golden and cooked through (you may need to do this in batches).

4. Heat the grill to medium-high. Pour the hot tomato sauce into an ovenproof dish, arrange the chicken on top of the sauce, top each chicken breast with mozzarella slices, then grill for 5 minutes until golden and bubbling.

5. Season well and scatter with basil leaves to serve.

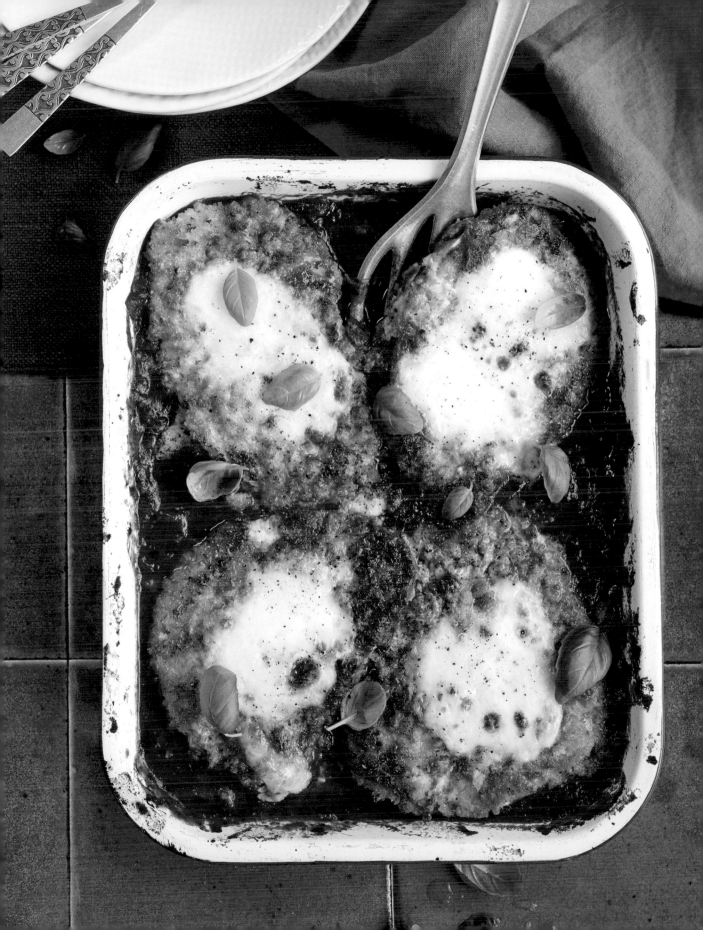

Speedy Chilli con Carne

Using a ready-made salsa means you won't need to add tomatoes, spices and flavourings separately. As an added bonus, it also reduces the cooking time.

Hands-on time: 10 minutes
Cooking time: about
   25 minutes
Serves 6

1 tbsp vegetable oil
1 onion, finely chopped
500g (1lb 2oz) lean beef mince
2 x 226g jars mild gluten-free
   tomato salsa
410g tin kidney beans, drained
   and rinsed
2 tbsp tomato purée
½ x 198g tin sweetcorn,
   drained
Large handful of fresh
   coriander (optional)

PER SERVING 416cals,
36g protein, 16g fat (6g
saturates), 34g carbs (19g
total sugars), 6g fibre

1. Put the vegetable oil in a large pan set over medium-high heat. Add the chopped onion and mince and fry them, breaking up the mince with a wooden spoon, for 10 minutes until the beef is well browned.

2. Stir in the salsa, kidney beans, tomato purée and sweetcorn, then bring to the boil. Simmer the chilli for 10–15 minutes until the mince is cooked through.

3. Remove from the heat and stir through the coriander, if using, then season to taste. Serve the chilli with freshly cooked rice or corn tortillas, or use as a filling for jacket potatoes.

● GH TIP
Check the salsa is gluten free if required.

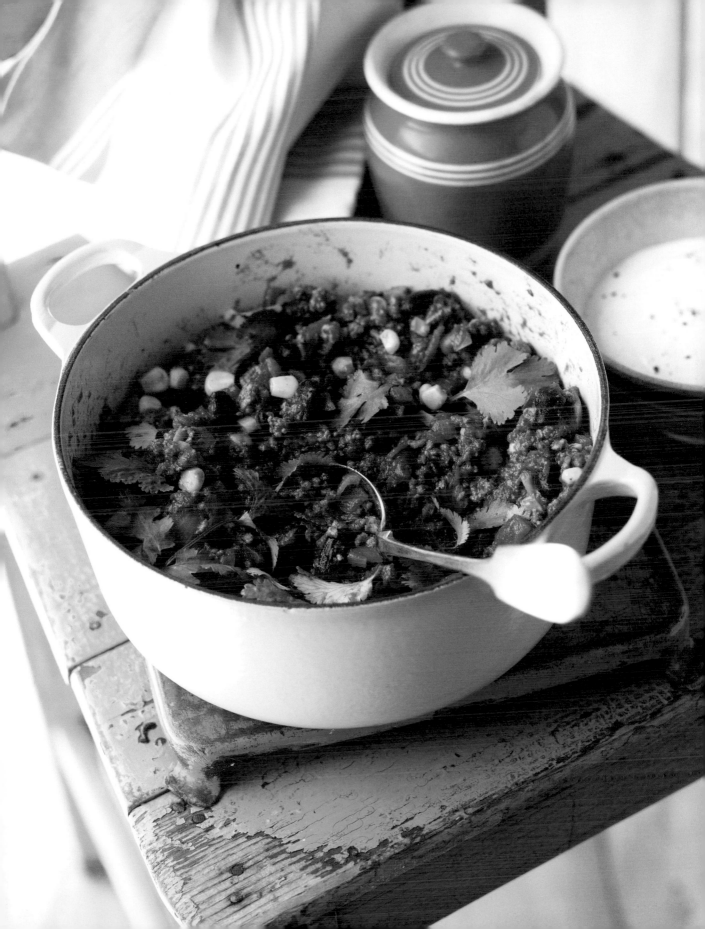

Chicken Satay Noodles

Nutty satay sauce, juicy chicken and a pile of noodles…
This dish ticks all the boxes for a flavourful, feel-good,
easy supper.

Hands-on time: 15 minutes
Cooking time: about
   15 minutes
Serves 4

1 tbsp vegetable oil
500g (1lb 2oz) chicken
   thigh fillets (skinless and
   boneless), cut into bite-
   sized pieces
½ tbsp ground coriander
3 tbsp medium curry paste
3 tbsp crunchy peanut butter
2 tbsp light brown soft sugar
165ml tin full-fat coconut milk
150g (5oz) sugar snap peas
200g (7oz) baby sweetcorn,
   chopped
Juice of 1 lemon
300g (11oz) fresh straight-to-
   wok egg noodles
Large handful of fresh
   coriander, roughly chopped

PER SERVING 615cals,
43g protein, 34g fat (11g
saturates), 33g carbs (12g
total sugars), 3g fibre

1. Heat the oil in a large wok or deep frying pan and fry the chicken
   for 8 minutes until it is golden and cooked through. Add the ground
   coriander and curry paste and fry for 1 minute more.

2. Stir in the peanut butter, sugar and coconut milk until well combined
   and bring to the boil. Add the sugar snap peas and sweetcorn and
   simmer for 3–4 minutes until the vegetables are just tender.

3. Stir in the lemon juice, then fold through the noodles and most of the
   coriander. Heat until the sauce and noodles are piping hot, adding a
   little water, if needed, to loosen the sauce. Season to taste, then divide
   among 4 bowls, sprinkle over the remaining coriander and serve.

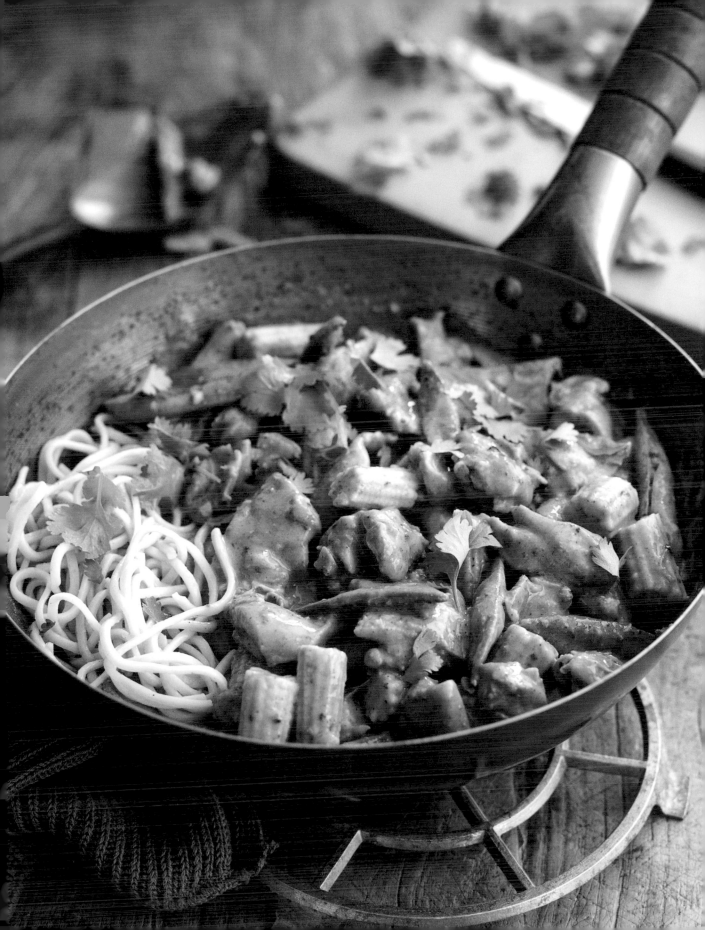

Salmon Pasta Bake

Part fish pie, part pasta bake, this hearty and tasty dish is quick to make, too. Use lightly smoked fish, if you like.

Hands-on time: 5 minutes
Cooking time: 20 minutes
Serves 4

75g (3oz) butter
75g (3oz) plain flour
900ml (1½ pints) milk
500g pack spinach and ricotta tortellini
150g (5oz) frozen peas
4 tbsp freshly chopped chives
375g (13oz) salmon fillets, skinned and cut into 2cm (¾in) pieces
50g (2oz) mature Cheddar cheese, grated

PER SERVING 761cals, 42g protein, 39g fat (19g saturates), 232g carbs (13g total sugars), 7g fibre

1. Preheat the oven to 200°C (180°C fan) mark 6. Melt the butter in a large pan over a medium heat and add the flour. Cook, stirring, for 30 seconds, then take the mixture off the heat and gradually stir in the milk. Return the pan to the heat and cook, stirring constantly, until the sauce is thickened.

2. Add the tortellini to the pan and bubble for 1 minute. Take the pan off the heat and fold through the peas, most of the chives, the salmon and plenty of seasoning.

3. Empty the mixture into an ovenproof serving dish and scatter over the cheese and remaining chives. Cook in the oven for 20 minutes or until bubbling and golden. Serve with a crisp green salad.

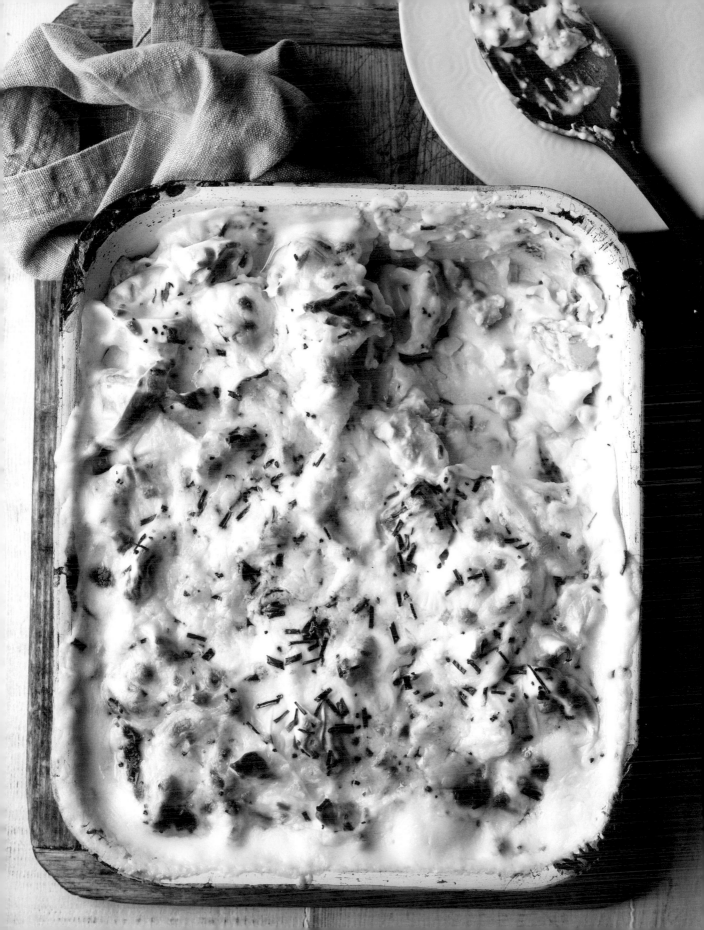

Fig, Parma Ham and Dolcelatte Pizza

It's hard to beat homemade pizza when you're craving comfort food, and this grown-up version turns it into a special meal.

Hands-on time: 15 minutes
Cooking time: 15 minutes
Serves 4

300g (11oz) strong white flour, plus extra to dust
7g sachet fast-action dried yeast
1 tsp caster sugar
1 tsp fine salt
2 tbsp extra virgin olive oil

FOR THE TOPPING
200g (7oz) Dolcelatte cheese
8 slices Parma ham, about 90g (3¼oz)
6 figs, quartered
50g (2oz) walnut pieces
Handful of rocket, to serve

PER SERVING (½ pizza)
697cals, 30g protein, 35g fat (14g saturates), 62g carbs (10g total sugars), 5g fibre

1. In a large bowl, mix together the flour, yeast, sugar and salt. Quickly stir in the oil and 175ml (6fl oz) lukewarm water to make a rough dough. Tip the dough on to a floured work surface and knead it for a few minutes. Form it into a rough ball, then cover the dough with the upturned bowl and leave it to rise for 5 minutes.

2. Preheat the oven to 220°C (200°C fan) mark 7. Re-flour your work surface and divide the dough in half. Roll out each piece into a 30.5cm (12in) base. Transfer each base to a baking sheet lined with baking paper.

3. Dot small spoonfuls of the Dolcelatte evenly over the bases, leaving a 1.5cm (⅔in) border of dough. Rip the ham slices in half lengthways and arrange on the bases. Dot over the fig quarters and scatter over the walnuts. Season the pizzas with freshly ground black pepper, then cook in oven for 12–15 minutes until golden.

4. Top each pizza with some rocket and serve in slices.

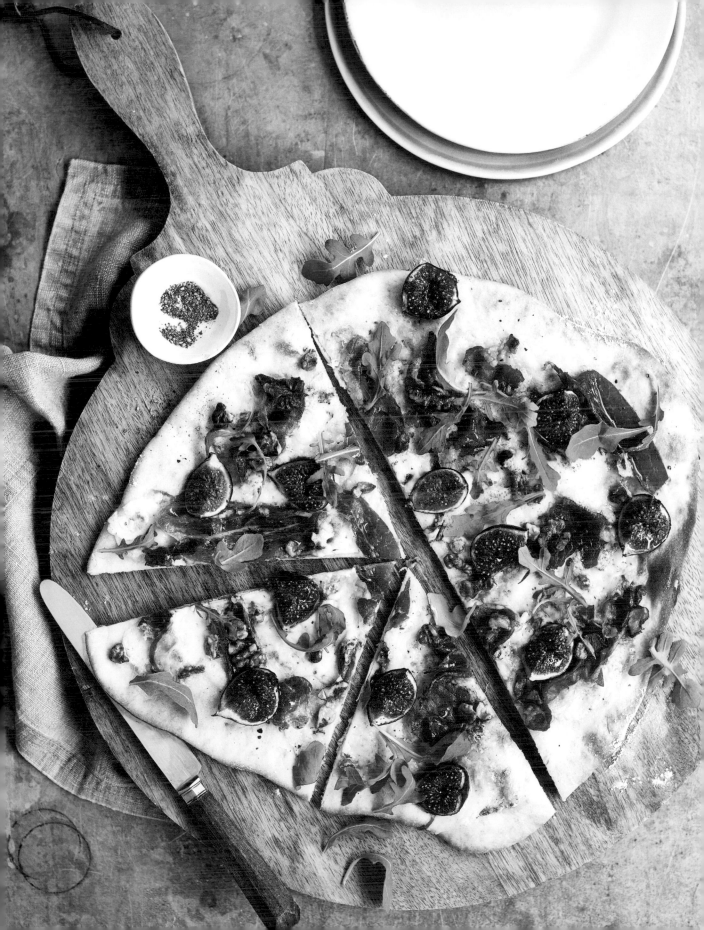

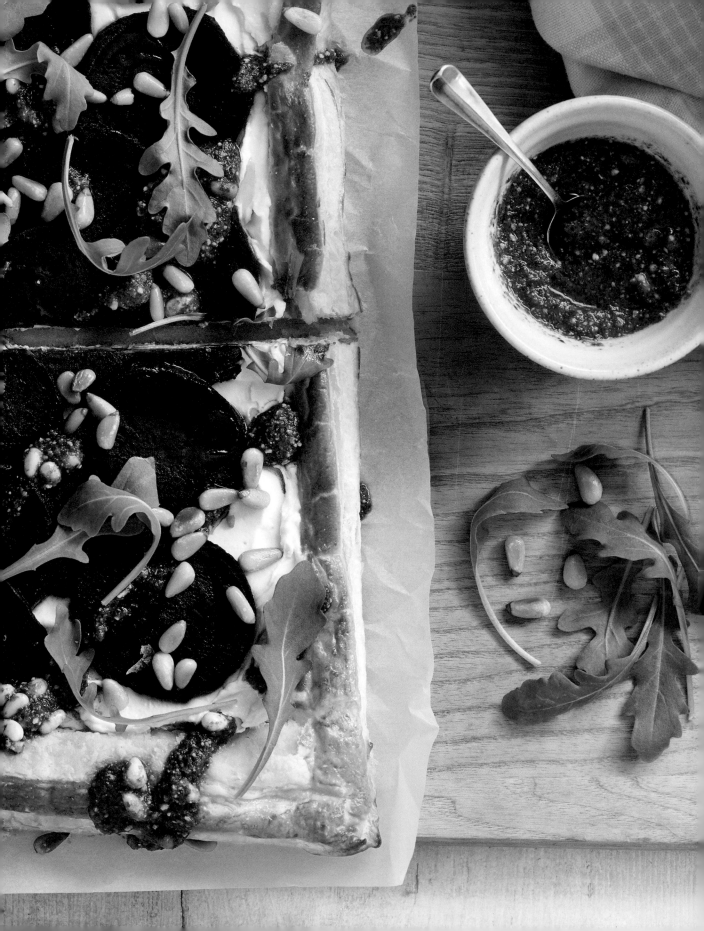

Speedy
Entertaining

Beet and Pinenut Hummus Salad

We've used a mix of normal and pink-striped candy beetroot to give this unique salad added wow-factor. Delicious 'hummus' made from pinenuts rather than traditional chickpeas makes this really special.

Hands-on time: 20 minutes, plus soaking
Serves 6

4 small to medium raw beetroots
Large handful of rocket
2 large oranges, peeled and cut into segments (reserve any juice)
Olive oil, to drizzle (optional)

FOR THE PINENUT HUMMUS
100g pack pinenuts
1 courgette, roughly chopped
Juice of 1 lemon
1 small garlic clove, crushed
1 tbsp tahini
2 tbsp extra virgin olive oil

PER SERVING 233cals, 6g protein, 17g fat (2g saturates), 11g carbs (11g total sugars), 4g fibre

1. Put the pinenuts into a bowl and cover with cold water. Leave them to soak for 15 minutes.

2. Wearing gloves to prevent your hands from staining, peel the beetroots and slice into 5mm (¼in) rounds. Arrange in a single layer on kitchen paper.

3. Drain the pinenuts and empty them into a food processor with the remaining hummus ingredients and some seasoning. Whiz to combine.

4. To serve, arrange the beetroot slices on a large platter or board. Pipe or spoon a dollop of hummus on to each slice. Scatter over the rocket and orange segments, then drizzle over some of the reserved orange juice and oil, if using.

◆ GET AHEAD
Make the pinenut 'hummus' up to a day ahead, cover and chill. Slice the beetroot up to an hour ahead of time and leave on kitchen paper. Complete the recipe to serve.

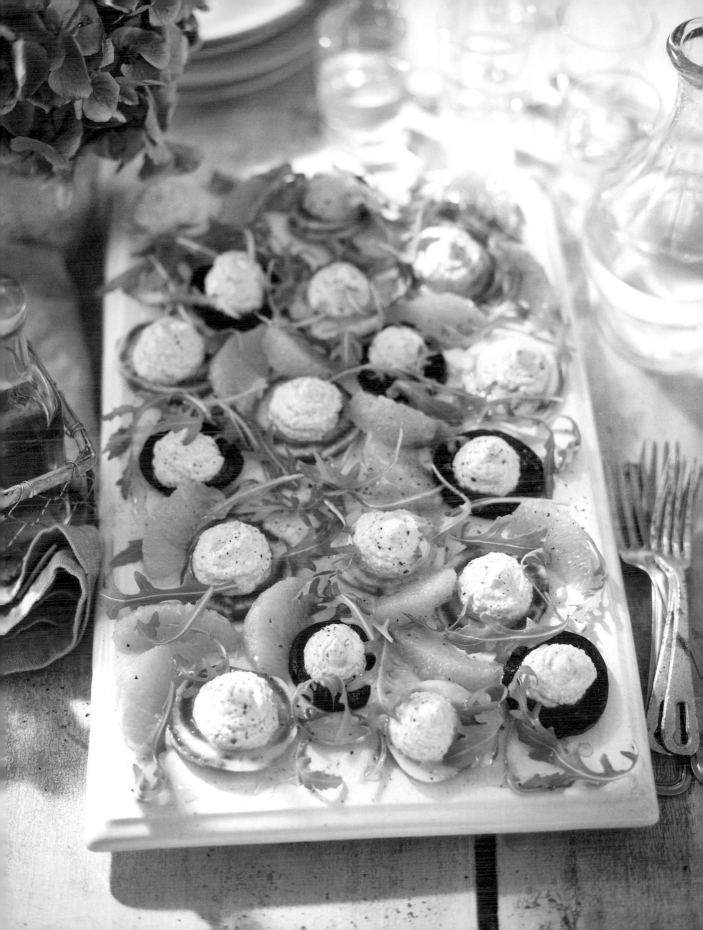

BRUSCHETTA BAR

These DIY starters are just the ticket when friends come round.

Ciabatta Toasts

Use these as a base for bruschetta or serve with your favourite cheese or pâté.

Cut a loaf of ciabatta into 18 x 2.5cm (1in) slices. Brush both sides of each slice with olive oil and toast them in batches on a hot griddle pan for 2 minutes on each side, until charred and crisp.

◆ GET AHEAD
Griddle the toasts up to 2 hours ahead of serving.

Goat's Cheese, Parma Ham and Basil Drizzle Bruschetta

Hands-on time: 10 minutes
Cooking time: about
   10 minutes
Serves 6

6 Parma ham slices
Large handful of fresh basil
   leaves
4 tbsp olive oil
Squeeze of lemon juice
75g (3oz) soft goat's cheese
18 Ciabatta Toasts (see box,
   above)

PER SERVING (3 toasts)
172cals, 7g protein, 12g fat
(4g saturates), 8g carbs (1g
total sugars), 1g fibre

1. Fry the ham slices in a hot pan for 1–2 minutes on each side until crispy and golden. Set aside on kitchen paper.

2. In a food processor, whiz the basil leaves, olive oil and a squeeze of lemon juice until the mixture is as smooth as you can get it.

3. Serve the goat's cheese, crispy Parma ham and ciabatta toasts on a platter with basil oil on the side to drizzle over.

◆ GET AHEAD
Cook the Parma ham up to 2 hours ahead. Make the basil oil up to 1 hour ahead. Complete the recipe to serve.

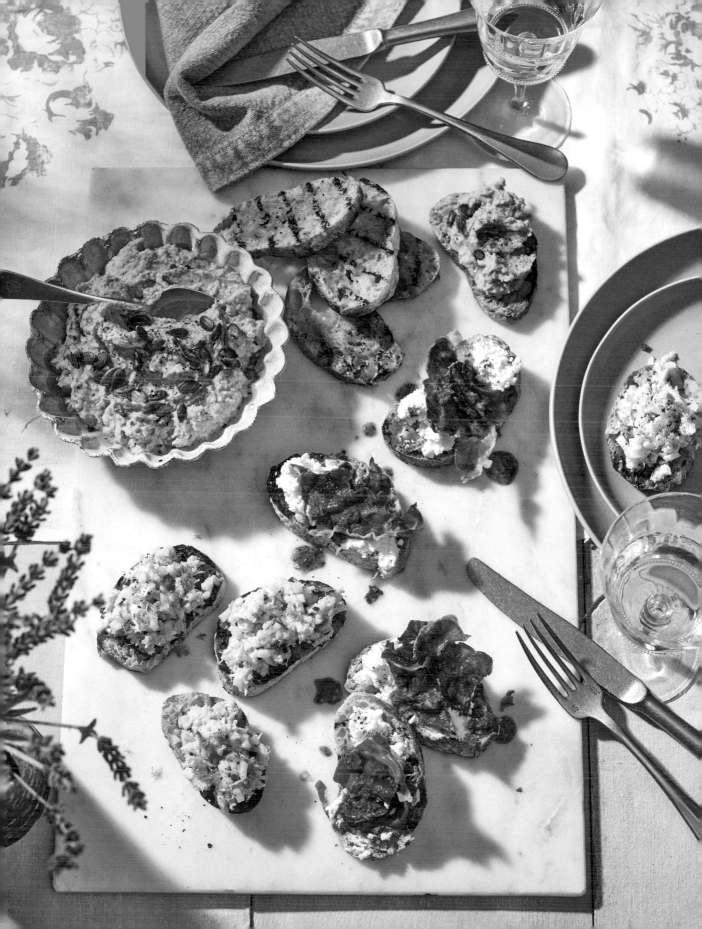

Crab, Fennel and Chilli Bruschetta

Hands-on time: 5 minutes
Serves 6

200g (7oz) white crabmeat
Finely grated zest of 1 lemon
1 tbsp olive oil
1 small fennel bulb, finely
  diced (keep the fennel
  fronds for garnish)
½–1 red chilli, deseeded and
  finely chopped, to taste
18 Ciabatta Toasts (see box on
  page 228)

PER SERVING (3 toasts)
109cals, 9g protein, 4g fat
(1g saturates), 8g carbs
(1g total sugars), 1g fibre

1. In a bowl, mix the crabmeat, lemon zest, olive oil and diced fennel with some seasoning and chopped red chilli, to taste. Cover and chill until needed.

2. To serve, remove the crabmeat mixture from the fridge, stir well and transfer to a bowl. Spoon onto ciabatta toasts to serve.

◆ GET AHEAD
Make the crabmeat mixture up to a day ahead. Cover and chill. To serve, stir the crabmeat mixture well and complete the recipe.

Roasted Carrot Hummus Bruschetta

Hands-on time: 10 minutes
Cooking time: 25 minutes
Serves 6

300g (11oz) carrots, thinly
  sliced into 5mm rounds
1 tbsp olive oil, plus extra to
  drizzle
400g tin chickpeas, drained
  and rinsed
3 tbsp tahini
3 tbsp lemon juice, plus extra
  to taste
3 tbsp olive oil
2 garlic cloves, crushed
1½ tsp ground cumin
Handful of pumpkin seeds
18 Ciabatta Toasts (see box on
  page 228)

PER SERVING 232 cals,
7g protein, 14g fat
(2g saturates), 18g carbs
(4g total sugars), 6g fibre

1. Heat the oven to 220°C (200°C fan) mark 7. Toss the carrots in a large roasting tin with the olive oil and some seasoning. Spread out in a single layer. Cover tightly with foil and cook in the oven for 10 minutes. Remove the foil, turn and roast for a further 15 minutes until tender and golden.

2. Remove the tray from the oven and empty the roast carrots into a food processor. Add the chickpeas, tahini, lemon juice, olive oil, crushed garlic, cumin and a splash of water, then whiz until the hummus is smooth. Check the seasoning, adding a little water to thin the mixture or lemon juice to sharpen it.

3. Transfer the hummus to a bowl, drizzle with a little extra olive oil and sprinkle over the pumpkin seeds. Serve with the ciabatta toasts on the side for dipping.

◆ GET AHEAD
Make the hummus up to 2 days ahead. Cover and chill. Remove the hummus from the fridge 1 hour before serving – you may want to stir through a little more olive oil to loosen it. Complete the recipe to serve.

Blinis with Whipped Goat's Cheese and Honey

These little bites are easy to assemble, and using ready-made blinis saves even more time. If you're not a fan of goat's cheese, use plain cream cheese instead.

Hands-on time: 15 minutes
Makes 24 canapés

150g (5oz) soft goat's cheese
4 tbsp double cream
Small bunch each of mint
   and parsley, leaves finely
   chopped
Zest of ½ lemon
24 ready-made blinis
Runny honey

PER CANAPÉ 59cals,
2g protein, 4g fat
(2g saturates), 3g carbs
(0g total sugars), 0.2g fibre

1. Using a hand-held electric whisk, whip the goat's cheese until light, then whisk in the double cream. Fold in the finely chopped herbs, lemon zest and some seasoning.

2. Top each ready-made blini with a dollop of the cheese mixture, then drizzle with runny honey and serve.

Radish with Creamy Cheese and Basil Dip

Fresh basil and creamy cheese make the perfect accompaniment for crisp, peppery radishes.

Hands-on time: 5 minutes
Serves 8

5 tbsp finely grated pecorino-
    style vegetarian hard cheese
2 tbsp fresh basil, chopped
Zest of 1 lemon
280g tub full-fat cream cheese
2 tbsp soured cream
100g bag ready-made olive oil
    crostini
500g (1lb 2oz) bunch radishes,
    washed thoroughly

PER SERVING 191cals,
5g protein, 14g fat (8g
saturates), 11g carbs (3g
total sugars), 1g fibre

1. Put the pecorino-style cheese, basil, lemon zest, cream cheese, soured cream and a generous grinding of black pepper into a small food processor. Whiz until the mixture is smooth, then transfer to a small serving bowl.

2. Put the crostini into a food bag and seal. Bash with a rolling pin until it forms rough crumbs, then tip into a serving dish.

3. Serve the dip, crostini crumbs and radishes together on a platter.

◆ GET AHEAD
Keep the dip in an airtight container in the fridge for up to 4 hours before serving. Store the crostini crumbs in an airtight container at room temperature for up to 2 days.

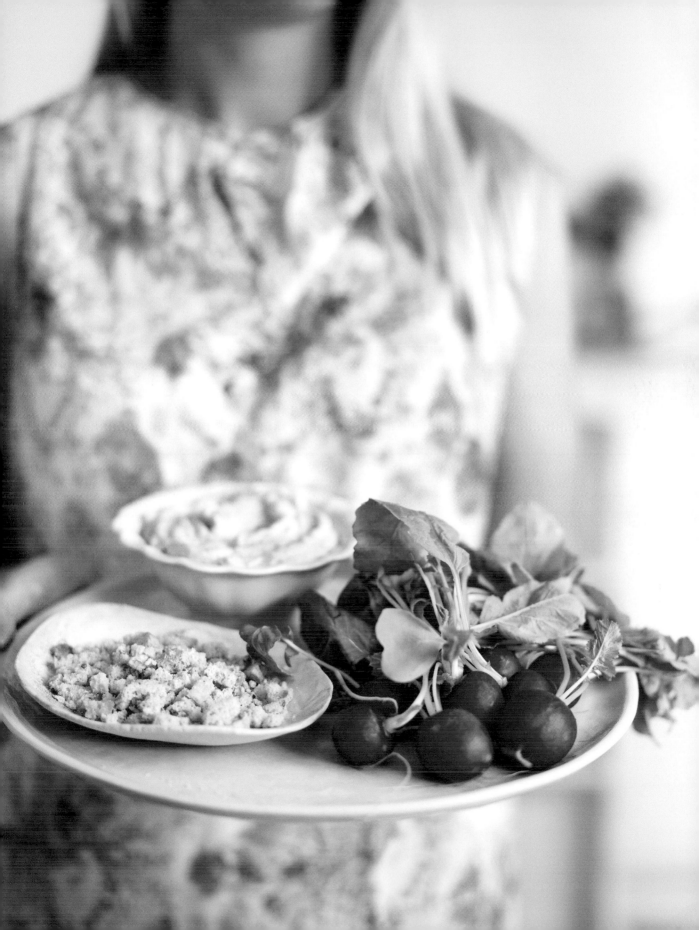

Fresh Vietnamese Prawn Rolls

These rolls are much lighter than the deep-fried variety and are perfect for using up leftover meats and vegetables.

Hands-on time: 30 minutes
Serves 4

150g (5oz) cooked straight-to-wok rice noodles
1 small carrot, grated
½ Little Gem lettuce, shredded
8 x 22cm (8½in) circular rice paper spring roll wrappers (available online from Thai and Vietnamese specialty stores)
Large handful of fresh mint leaves
200g (7oz) cooked and peeled king prawns
100g (3½oz) sweet chilli sauce
1 tbsp Thai fish sauce
2 tsp rice wine vinegar
2 courgettes, trimmed
25g (1oz) roasted salted peanuts, roughly chopped

PER SERVING 172cals, 16g protein, 5g fat (1g saturates), 17g carbs (7g total sugars), 2g fibre

1. Put the rice noodles in a large bowl and cover with boiling water from a kettle. Leave to soak for 3 minutes, drain in a sieve, then run the sieve under cold water to cool and refresh the noodles. Drain again and empty the noodles into a medium bowl. Add the carrot and lettuce and mix to combine.

2. Soak a rice paper wrapper according to the pack instructions, then lay on a board. Setting some mint leaves aside for the salad, arrange a few mint leaves and prawns in a strip across the centre of the circle, leaving a 2.5cm (1in) border at each end. Top with one-eighth of the noodle mixture. Fold the bottom of the wrapper up and over the filling, then fold in the sides before rolling up the wrapper to encase the filling. Repeat with the remaining wrappers – don't overfill the rolls or they will be difficult to seal. Transfer the rolls to a serving platter (seam-side down).

3. In a small bowl, stir together the sweet chilli sauce, fish sauce and rice vinegar. Using a y-shaped peeler, peel the courgettes into ribbons. Put them into a large bowl with the peanuts and remaining mint leaves. Add 3 tablespoons of the sweet chilli mixture and toss through to coat.

4. Serve the prawn rolls and salad with the remaining sauce on the side.

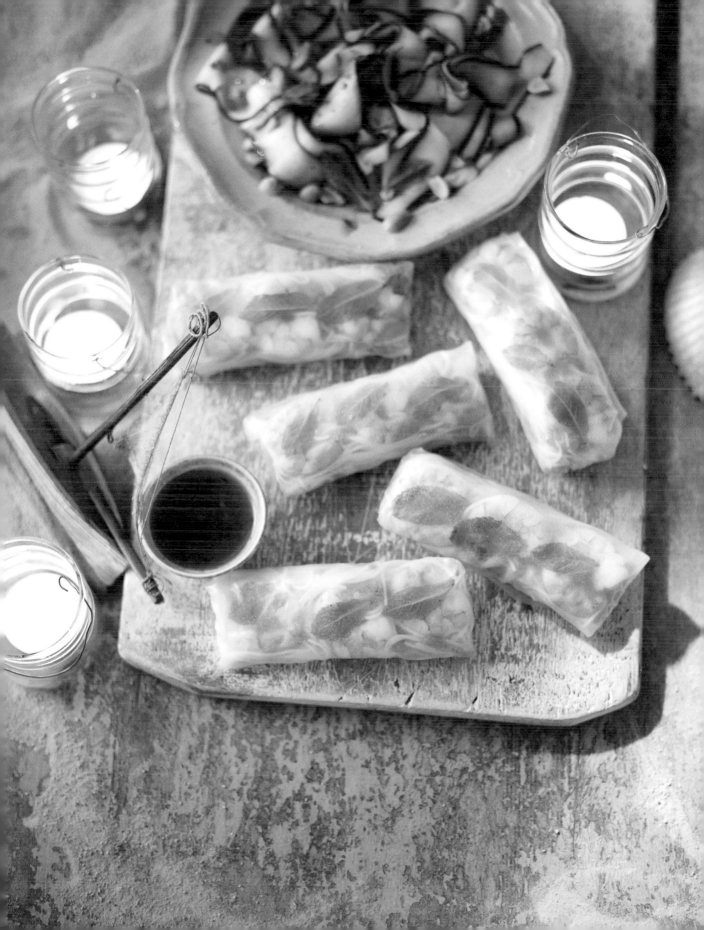

Pint O'Prawn and Smoked Salmon Cocktail

Prawn cocktail gets an update with the addition of hot smoked salmon. Served pub-style with crusty bread this makes a fun starter or light lunch.

**Hands-on time: 15 minutes
Serves 4**

2 fillets hot-smoked salmon,
  skinned and flaked
2 x 150g packs cooked and
  peeled king prawns
3 avocados, peeled, stoned
  and chopped
Juice of 1 lemon
4 Little Gem lettuces, trimmed
  and chopped
Crusty bread, to serve

FOR THE MARIE ROSE
  SAUCE
6 tbsp mayonnaise
3 tbsp ketchup
Pinch of paprika, to taste
Dash of Tabasco, to taste

**PER SERVING 573cals,
36g protein, 43g fat (8g
saturates), 7g carbs (6g total
sugars), 6g fibre**

1. In a medium bowl, mix together the mayonnaise and ketchup for the Marie Rose sauce, adding the paprika, Tabasco and some seasoning, to taste. Spoon half the sauce into a little bowl to serve alongside the seafood cocktail.

2. Add the hot-smoked salmon and a third of the prawns to the remaining sauce and mix together. Divide the mixture among 4 pint glasses or serving glasses.

3. In a clean medium-size bowl, toss the avocados in lemon juice. Add the remaining prawns and the lettuce and toss together.

4. Add a layer of avocado prawns to each of the serving glasses. Serve with the reserved Marie Rose sauce and crusty bread.

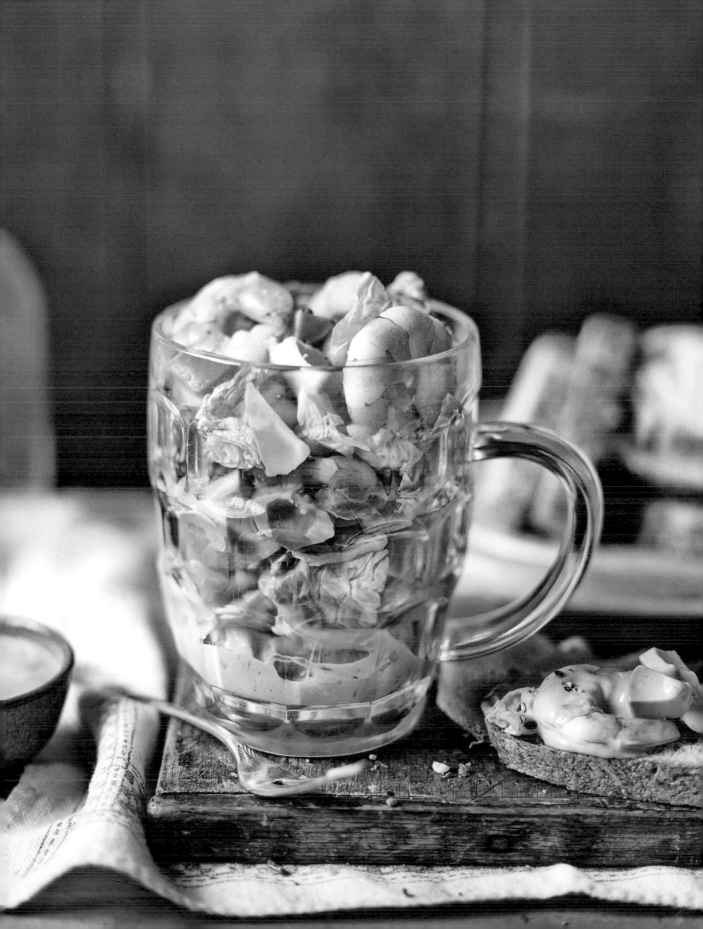

Cider and Tarragon Mussels

Sustainable and great value, mussels make a delicious midweek meal. As the old adage goes, they're in season when there's an 'R' in the month – roughly from September through to April. This dish can be made with clams, too, for an elegant dinner-party starter.

Hands-on time: 5 minutes
Cooking time: 15 minutes
Serves 4

2kg (4½lb) prepared mussels
25g (1oz) ready-made garlic butter, plus extra to serve (optional)
1 tbsp olive oil
3 large shallots, finely sliced
500ml (17fl oz) dry cider
200ml (⅓ pint) vegetable or fish stock
Handful of fresh tarragon leaves, chopped
Crusty bread, toasted, to serve (optional)

PER SERVING 501cals,
61g protein, 22g fat (9g saturates), 5g carbs (5g total sugars), 1g fibre

1. Sort through the mussels to remove any open ones, then clean the closed mussels under running water, removing any barnacles and beards with a cutlery knife. Firmly tap any open mussels – if they close, they are fine to use, but any that remain open should be discarded.

2. Melt the garlic butter and oil in a very large pan with a tight-fitting lid set over medium heat. Add the shallots and cook for 10 minutes until soft.

3. Increase the heat, pour in the cider and stock, then cover and bring to the boil. Tip in the mussels and cover again. Simmer for 5 minutes, shaking occasionally, until the mussels have fully opened (discard any that remain closed).

4. Stir through most of the tarragon and divide the mussels among 4 bowls, then sprinkle over the remaining tarragon. Serve with toasted bread spread with garlic butter, if you like.

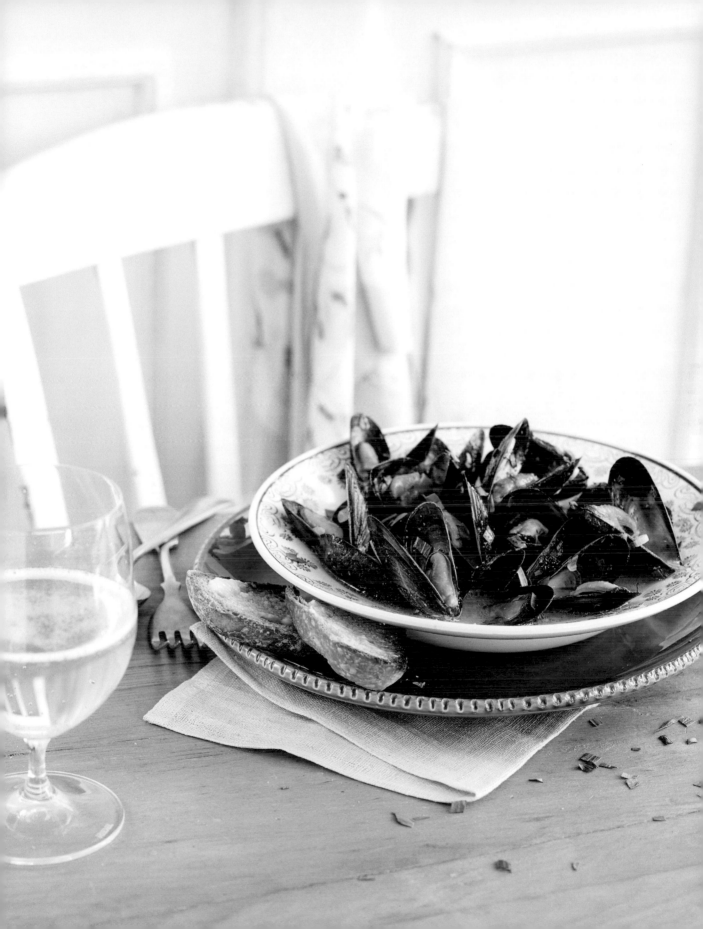

Watermelon 'Steak' Salad

Use a metal skewer to poke out seeds from the watermelon slices. Serve with toasted pitta breads on the side, if you like.

Hands-on time: 20 minutes
Serves 4

100g (3 oz) rocket
50g (2oz) pitted black olives, roughly chopped
50g (2oz) pumpkin or sunflower seeds
1 red onion, finely chopped
40g (1½oz) pistachio kernels, roughly chopped
2 tbsp freshly chopped fresh mint
2kg (4lb) whole watermelon
150g (5oz) goat's cheese or vegetarian feta
Pitta breads, to serve (optional)

FOR THE DRESSING
1 tsp Dijon mustard
1 small garlic clove, crushed
1 tsp caster sugar
3 tbsp extra virgin olive oil

PER SERVING 456cals, 15g protein, 32g fat (10g saturates), 25g carbs (23g total sugars), 3g fibre

1. In a small bowl, mix together all the dressing ingredients. Season and set aside.

2. In a large bowl, toss together the rocket, olives, pumpkin and sunflower seeds, onion, pistachios and mint. Set aside.

3. Leaving the skin on, cut 4 x 2.5cm (1in) slices from the mid-section of the watermelon (use any leftover watermelon for a fruit salad). Cut the skin off each slice so you are left with watermelon 'steaks', then pick out and discard the black seeds.

4. Chop or break up the goat's cheese or feta into bite-size pieces. Add to the rocket bowl with the dressing and toss together. Put a watermelon steak on to each plate and top with the rocket salad. Serve with toasted pitta bread on the side, if you like.

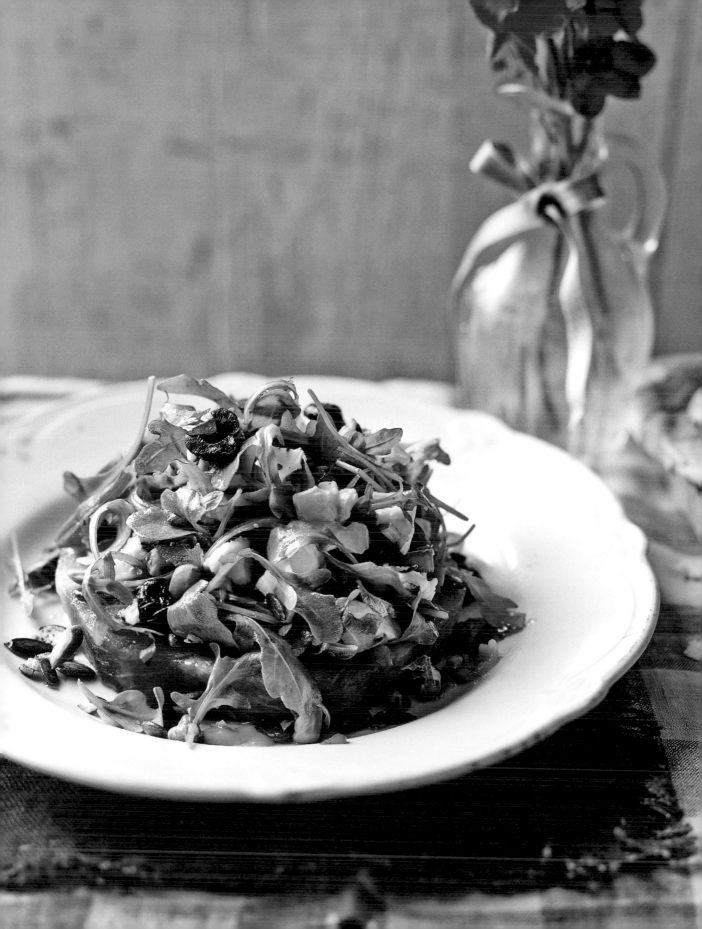

Beetroot and Goat's Cheese Puff Pastry Tart

Ready-rolled puff pastry keeps for a few weeks in the fridge and is perfect for whipping up an impromptu tart.

Hands-on time: 5 minutes
Cooking time: about
 25 minutes
Serves 4

320g pack ready-rolled all-
 butter puff pastry
1 medium egg, beaten
2 x 125g packs soft goat's
 cheese
100g (3½oz) cream cheese
250g pack pre-cooked
 beetroot (in natural juices),
 drained and cut into thin
 rounds
3 tbsp fresh basil pesto
2 tbsp pinenuts, toasted
Small handful of rocket

PER SERVING 690cals,
 22g protein, 53g fat (30g
 saturates), 32g carbs (3g
 total sugars), 1g fibre

1. Preheat the oven to 220°C (200°C fan) mark 7. Line a large baking tray with baking paper. Unroll the pastry and lift the sheet on to the lined tray. Use a knife to score a 1.5cm (⅔in) border around the edge of the pastry (do not cut all the way through). Brush the border with some beaten egg. Cook in the oven for 20 minutes.

2. Meanwhile, put the goat's cheese and cream cheese in a bowl and beat until light and fluffy, about 3 minutes.

3. Carefully remove the tray from the oven and, with the back of a spoon, gently press down the pastry inside the border. Spread the goat's cheese over the pastry, making sure to stay within the border, then top with the sliced beetroot. Return to the oven for a further 5 minutes. Remove from the oven and spoon over the pesto, then scatter over the toasted pinenuts and rocket and serve.

● GH TIP
Swap the pinenuts for walnuts, if you like.

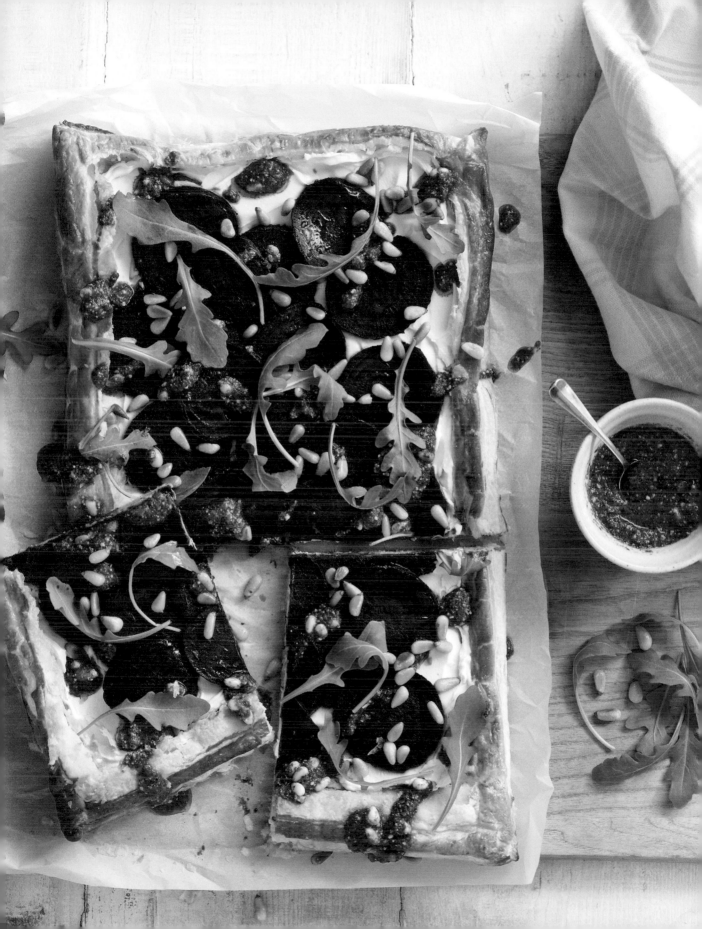

Fig and Parma Ham Salad

You can adapt this recipe with seasonal fruit – try it with ripe peaches or nectarines during the summer months or juicy ripe pears in autumn.

Hands-on time: 10 minutes
Serves 4

140g bag rocket, watercress
  and spinach leaves
6 ripe figs, quartered
8 slices Parma ham
2 balls buffalo mozzarella,
  drained
2 tbsp balsamic glaze
A few leaves of fresh mint
1 ciabatta loaf, sliced into
  chunks
1 tsp olive oil, to brush
1 garlic clove, peeled

PER SERVING 452cals,
27g protein, 20g fat (10g
saturates), 41g carbs (9g
total sugars), 4g fibre

1. On a large serving dish, arrange the salad leaves, figs and Parma ham. Tear the mozzarella into small pieces and dot among the salad. Drizzle over the balsamic glaze and garnish with the mint.

2. Meanwhile, toast the ciabatta until golden, then brush lightly with oil and rub the surface with garlic. Serve alongside the salad.

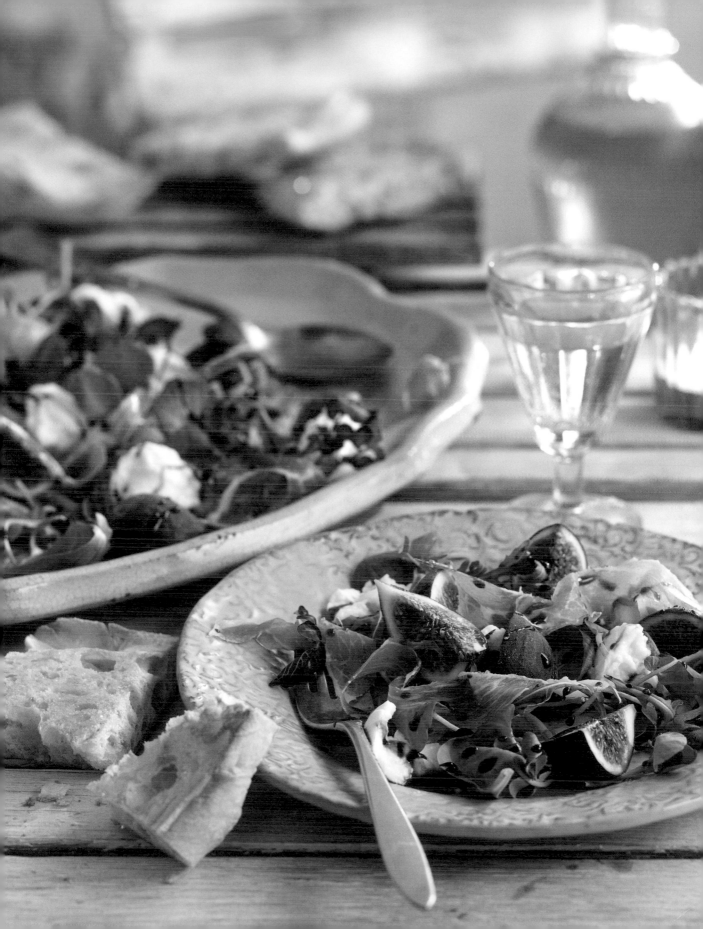

Squid and Chorizo Salad

Squid cooks very quickly, so it's ideal when you want to whip up a fast starter. Use scallops instead of squid, or fresh roasted peppers instead of roasted peppers from a jar, if you like.

Hands-on time: 10 minutes
Cooking time: about
   10 minutes
Serves 2

75g (3oz) gluten-free cooking
   chorizo, sliced into rounds
150g (5oz) prepared squid
   tubes, sliced into 1cm (½in)
   wide rings
4 tbsp sherry vinegar
1 tbsp caster sugar
1 shallot, finely sliced
50g (2oz) mild roasted
   peppers, from a jar
50g (2oz) watercress, to serve

PER SERVING 227cals,
20g protein, 12g fat (4g
saturates), 11g carbs (9g
total sugars), 1g fibre

1. Set a small frying pan over high heat and fry the chorizo for about 2 minutes until beginning to crisp and release its oil. Lift the chorizo out of the pan and into a bowl, leaving the chorizo oil in the pan. Add the squid to the pan and cook over high heat for 1–2 minutes until just cooked. Add to the chorizo bowl.

2. To the empty pan add the sherry vinegar, sugar and shallot and bubble for a few minutes until thickened. Meanwhile, cut the peppers in half.

3. Arrange the chorizo, squid, peppers and watercress on a platter. Drizzle over the sherry vinegar dressing and season well. Serve.

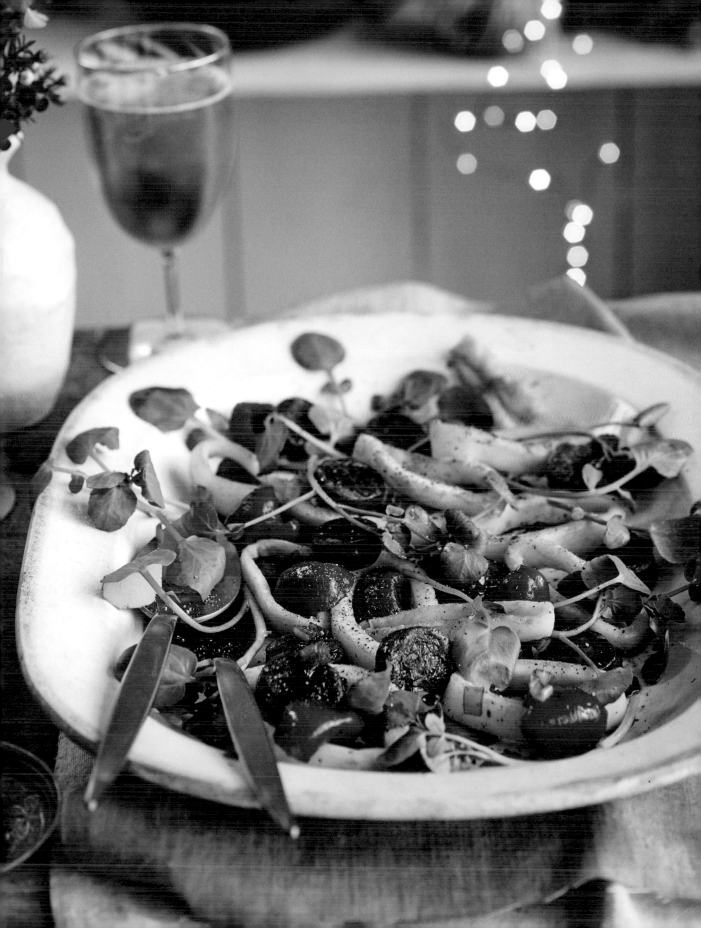

Sunday Lunch Salad

This dish borrows the ingredients of a classic roast and uses them to create a hearty salad for a summery twist on tradition.

Hands-on time: 10 minutes
Cooking time: about
   20 minutes
Serves 4

4 carrots, peeled and
   quartered lengthways
4 parsnips, peeled and
   quartered lengthways
3 tbsp sunflower oil
1 tbsp runny honey
Small head of cauliflower, cut
   into florets
50g (2oz) Cheddar cheese,
   grated
500g (1lb 2oz) sirloin steaks,
   fat trimmed and discarded
3 large cooked Yorkshire
   puddings, cut into 2cm
   (¾in) pieces
90g bag rocket

FOR THE HORSERADISH
   SAUCE
125g (4oz) crème fraîche
1 tbsp hot horseradish sauce
2 tbsp fresh parsley, finely
   chopped
½ tsp runny honey

PER SERVING 687cals,
42g protein, 36g fat (16g
saturates), 41g carbs (23g
total sugars), 15g fibre

1. Preheat the oven to 220°C (200°C fan) mark 7. In a large roasting tin, toss the carrots and parsnips with 1 tablespoon oil and the honey. Season well and roast for 20 minutes. In a small roasting tin, toss the cauliflower florets with another 1 tablespoon of oil and some seasoning, and roast for 15 minutes. Take the cauliflower out of the oven and sprinkle the cheese over the florets, then return to the oven for a further 5 minutes.

2. Meanwhile, heat the remaining 1 tablespoon of oil in a large frying pan. Season the steaks and fry for 2–3 minutes on each side, depending on how well you like your meat cooked. Remove the steaks from the pan to a board and leave to rest.

3. Scatter the Yorkshire pudding pieces on a baking tray and cook in the oven for 4–5 minutes until crispy.

4. In a small bowl, mix together the ingredients for the horseradish sauce with some seasoning and set aside. Thinly slice the steaks.

5. On a large platter, layer the rocket, roasted vegetables and beef. Top with the Yorkshire pudding croutons and serve warm with horseradish sauce.

● GH TIP
For a vegetarian-friendly version of this salad, omit the beef and add some raw beetroot wedges to the tin along with the carrots and parsnips.

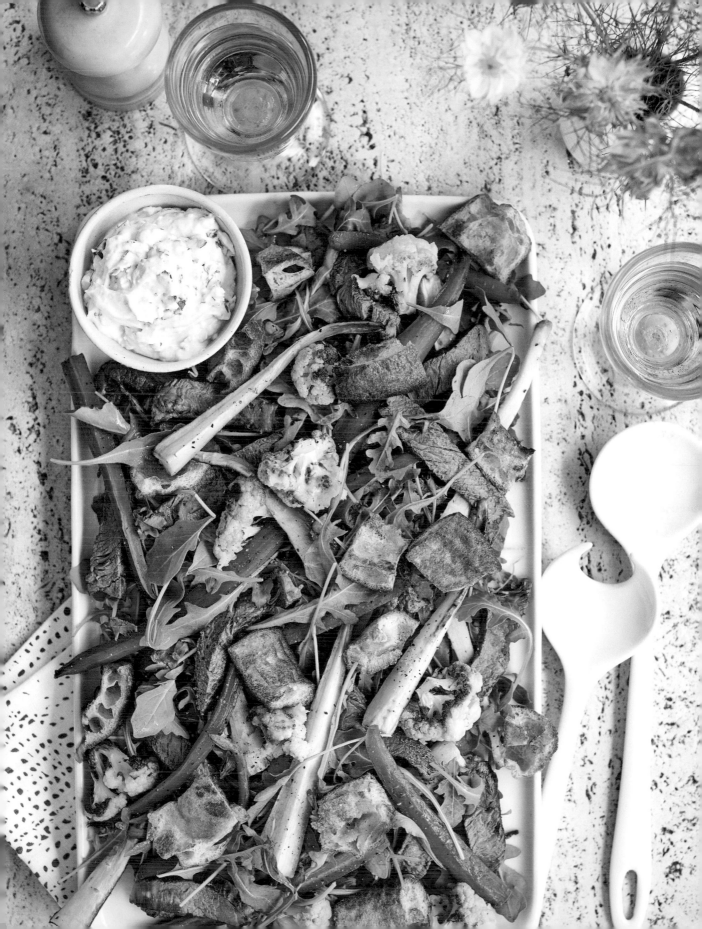

Curry Pork Steaks with Fruit Couscous

Couscous is one of the fastest grains to cook and goes well with full-flavoured food. As shoulder steaks are darker meat, they can still appear slightly pink when cooked – always check the meat is piping hot throughout.

Hands-on time: 10 minutes
Cooking time: 15 minutes
Serves 4

4 x 150g (5oz) pork shoulder
  steaks
2 tbsp medium-hot curry paste
150g (5oz) couscous
400g tin chickpeas, drained
  and rinsed
250ml (9fl oz) boiling chicken
  stock
75g (3oz) sultanas
Zest and juice of 1 lime
Large handful of fresh parsley,
  chopped
4 tsp aubergine (brinjal)
  pickle
Green salad, to serve

PER SERVING 718cals,
53g protein, 31g fat (9g
saturates), 53g carbs (16g
total sugars), 6g fibre

1. Heat the grill to high. Put the pork steaks on a board, cover with clingfilm and flatten slightly with a rolling pin. Transfer the steaks to a bowl, add the curry paste and plenty of seasoning and toss to coat the meat. Arrange the steaks on a non-stick baking tray, then grill for 12–13 minutes, turning once, until golden at the edges and cooked through.

2. Meanwhile, put the couscous and chickpeas in a large bowl and pour over the boiling stock. Cover with clingfilm and set aside for 5 minutes, then uncover and use a fork to fluff up the grains. Stir in the sultanas, lime zest and juice and most of the parsley.

3. When the pork is cooked through, spoon 1 teaspoon aubergine pickle on top of each steak, then garnish with the remaining parsley. Serve the pork with the couscous and a green salad.

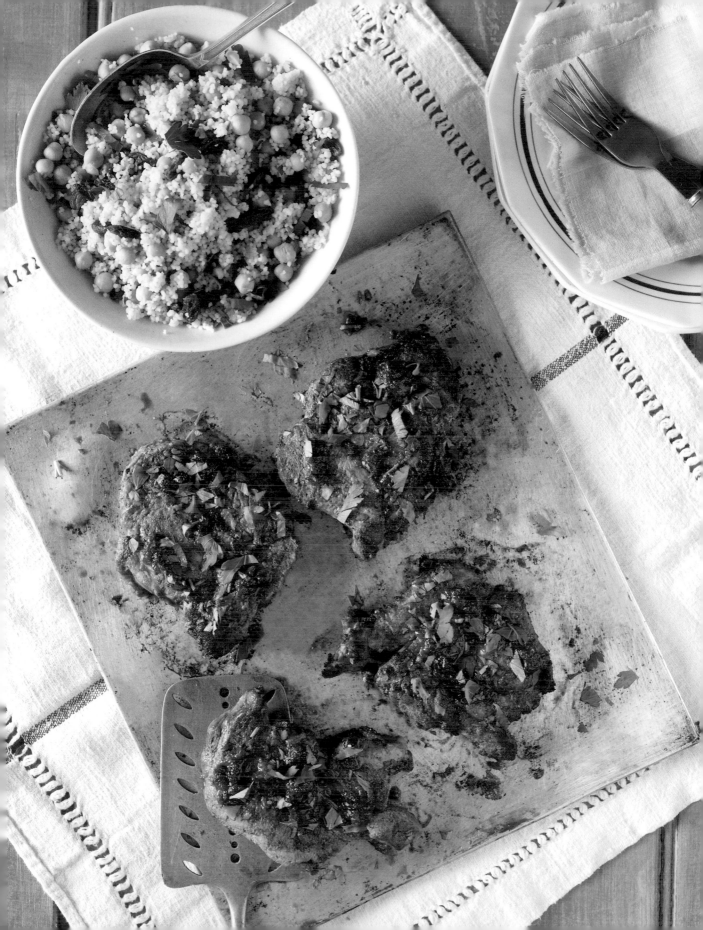

Steak with the Best Pan Sauce

The creamy, punchy sauce for this dish is made while the steak rests – so tasty, quick and easy!

Hands-on time: 15 minutes
Cooking time: about
    15 minutes
Serves 2

1 tbsp olive oil
15g (½oz) butter
2 beef steaks – fillet, rump or
   sirloin, as you prefer
100g (3½oz) chestnut
   mushrooms, sliced
4 smoked streaky bacon
   rashers, sliced
2 tbsp brandy (optional)
½ tbsp gluten-free wholegrain
   mustard
2 fresh thyme sprigs, leaves
   picked
125ml (4fl oz) double cream
Ready roasted potatoes and
   greens, to serve (optional)

PER SERVING 907cals,
64g protein, 68g fat (34g
saturates), 1g carbs (1g total
sugars), 1g fibre

1. Put the oil and butter in a medium frying pan set over medium-high heat. Pat the steaks dry with kitchen paper and season. When the butter is sizzling, fry the steaks for 4–5 minutes (depending on thickness) for medium meat, turning midway through. Cook the steaks for a slightly shorter or longer time if you prefer your meat rare or well done. Transfer the steaks to a board, cover with a few layers of foil and leave to rest at room temperature while you make the sauce.

2. To the empty pan, add the mushrooms and bacon and fry until the bacon is crisp and the mushrooms are tender. Add the brandy, if using, and bubble for 10 seconds. Stir in the mustard, thyme leaves and cream. Heat to warm everything through and check the seasoning. Serve the sauce with the rested steaks, with roasted potatoes and greens on the side, if you like.

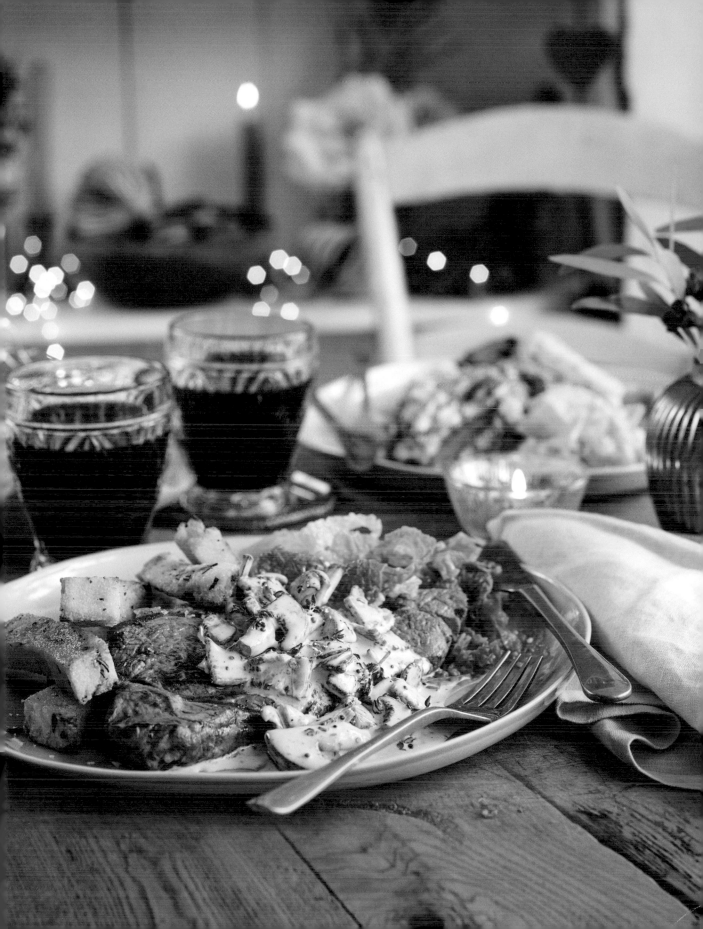

Rack of Lamb with Bean Salad

If you prefer, buy cutlets of lamb and brush the herb paste over them. Then grill for a couple of minutes on either side until cooked to your liking.

Hands-on time: 15 minutes
Cooking time: about 20
**   minutes**
Serves 4

50g (2oz) watercress
1 tbsp Dijon mustard
Large handful fresh parsley
Small handful fresh mint
    leaves
2 garlic cloves
1 tbsp olive oil
2 x 6-bone racks of lamb (fat
    removed, if you like)

FOR THE SALAD
2 x 400g tins mixed beans,
    drained and rinsed
½ red onion, finely chopped
2 tbsp fresh mint leaves, finely
    sliced
50–75g (2–3oz) feta cheese, to
    taste, crumbled
150g (5oz) cherry tomatoes,
    halved
1 tsp caster sugar
1 tbsp white wine vinegar

PER SERVING 565cals,
35g protein, 35g fat (15g
saturates), 25g carbs (5g
total sugars), 6g fibre

1. Preheat the oven to 200°C (180°C fan) mark 6. Put the watercress, mustard, herbs, garlic, oil and some seasoning into the small bowl of a food processor and whiz to a paste. Arrange the lamb racks on a baking sheet and spread the paste over the meaty side.

2. Roast the racks for 15–20 minutes for pink meat (or for longer or shorter as you prefer). Set aside to rest for 5 minutes.

3. Put all the salad ingredients into a bowl and fold together (trying not to break up the feta too much). Check the seasoning and set aside.

4. Once the lamb has rested, carve into cutlets and serve with the salad and seasonal vegetables, if you like.

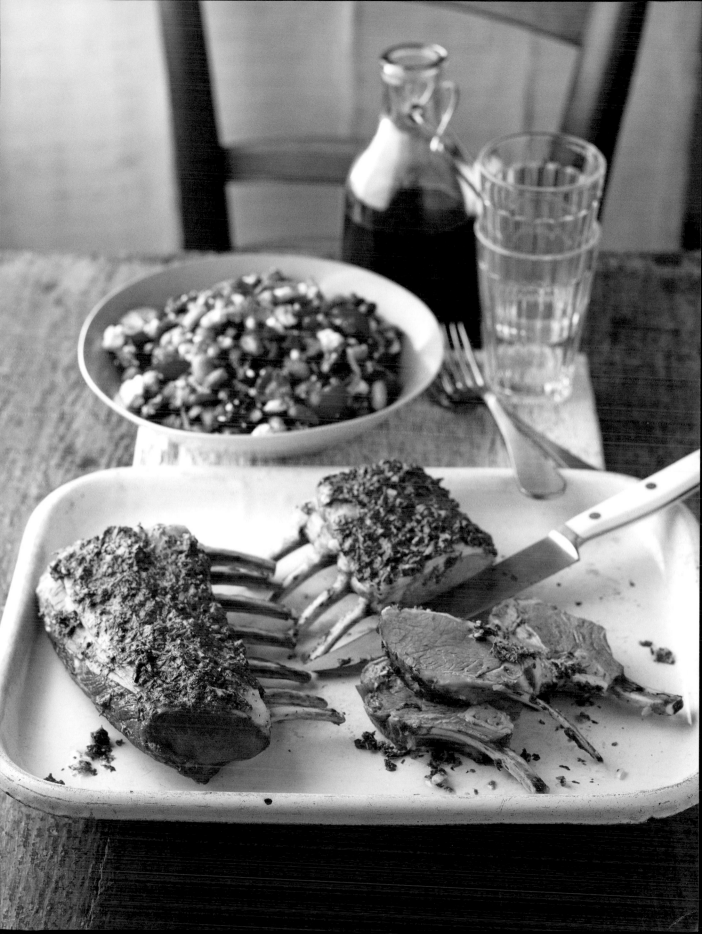

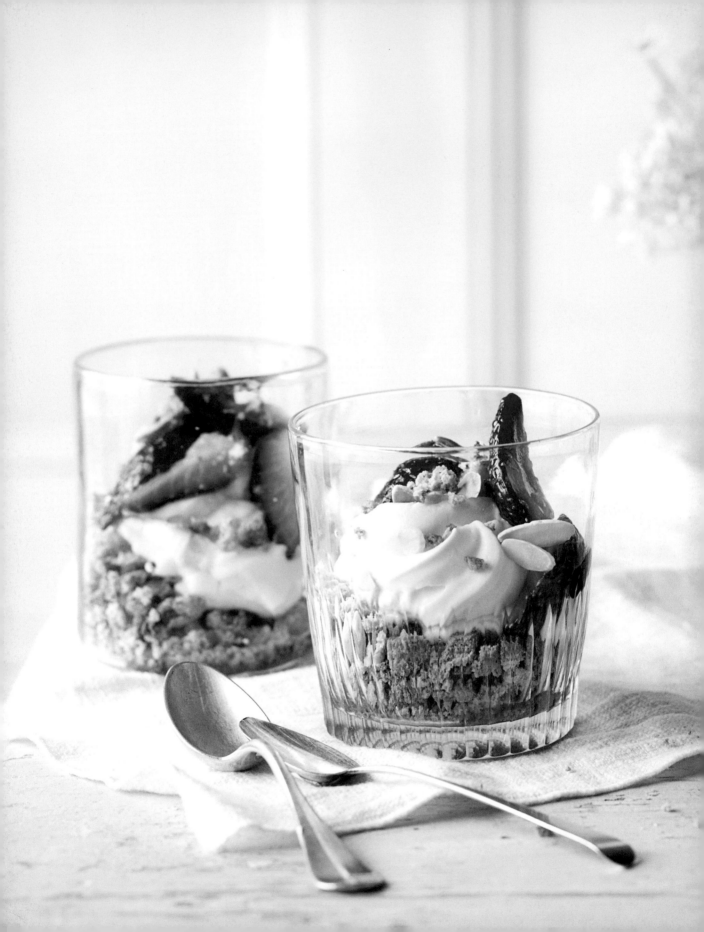

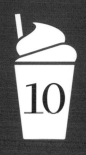

Sweet

MILKSHAKES

Hot weather? These indulgent ice-cream shakes are perfect for warm, balmy summer days – just the thing for a weekend treat or birthday celebration. Take your pick from fruity Raspberry Ripple, cool Choc-mint and moreish Peanut Butter Popcorn.

Raspberry Ripple

Hands-on time: 10 minutes
Makes 2 milkshakes

PER MILKSHAKE 350cals, 7g protein, 19g fat (11g saturates), 37g carbs (35g total sugars), 1g fibre

125g (4oz) raspberries, plus a few extra berries, to serve
2 tsp runny honey
4 large scoops vanilla ice cream
200ml (7fl oz) milk
Squirty cream, to decorate (optional)
Hundreds-and-thousands, to decorate (optional)

1. In a blender, whiz the raspberries and honey until smooth. Press the mixture through a sieve (discard the seeds). Rinse out the blender, then whiz together the ice cream and milk.

2. Drizzle some raspberry sauce into 2 tall glasses, then pour in the milkshake. Top each glass with more raspberry sauce, a few raspberries and some squirty cream and hundreds-and-thousands, if you like.

Choc-mint

Hands-on time: 10 minutes
Makes 2 milkshakes

PER MILKSHAKE (with cream, without toppings) 277cals, 7g protein, 18g fat (11g saturates), 23g carbs (22g total sugars), 0g fibre

4 large scoops mint chocolate ice cream
250ml (9fl oz) milk
Chocolate sauce, to serve
Squirty cream, to serve
1 small bar Mint Aero, to decorate (optional)
A chocolate wafer, to decorate (optional)

1. In a blender, whiz together the ice cream and milk.

2. Drizzle some chocolate sauce into 2 tall glasses, then pour in the milkshake. Top each glass with squirty cream, more chocolate sauce, some chopped Mint Aero and a chocolate wafer to finish, if you like.

Peanut Butter Popcorn

Hands-on time: 10 minutes
Makes 2 milkshakes

PER MILKSHAKE (with cream, without toppings) 466cals, 15g protein, 34g fat (14g saturates), 25g carbs (22g total sugars), 0g fibre

4 large scoops vanilla ice cream
250ml (9fl oz) milk
4 tbsp peanut butter
Small handful of toffee-flavour popcorn
Squirty cream, to serve
Reese's Peanut Butter Cups, to decorate (optional)
Caramel sauce, to serve (optional)

1. In a blender, whiz together the ice cream, milk, peanut butter and half of the toffee-flavour popcorn.

2. Pour the milkshake into 2 tall glasses. Top each with squirty cream, a little more popcorn, and some chopped Reese's Peanut Butter Cups and caramel sauce, if you like.

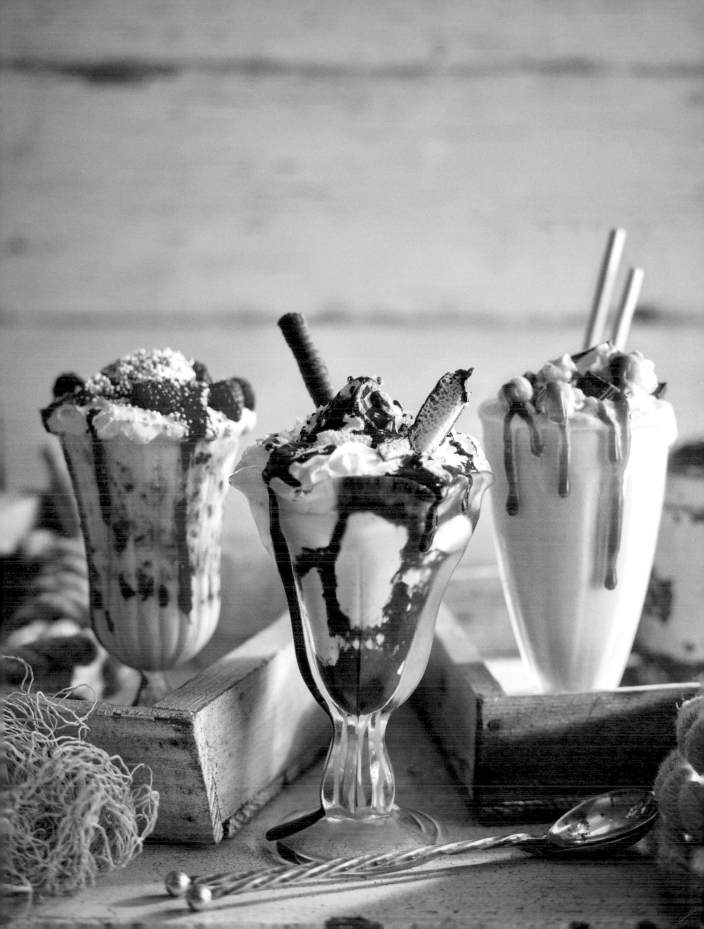

Black Forest Pots

So simple to make, these clever puds use ready-made brownies as a shortcut, but of course you can use homemade ones if you prefer. Tinned cherries are a brilliant storecupboard staple.

**Hands-on time: 10 minutes
Serves 6**

2 x 425g tins cherries, drained
4 tbsp cherry jam
300ml (½ pint) double cream
1 tbsp kirsch or amaretto
1 tbsp icing sugar
100g (3½ oz) brownies or
    brownie bites, crumbled,
    plus extra pieces to
    decorate
Small bar of dark chocolate,
    grated, to serve

PER SERVING 439cals,
2g protein, 32g fat (19g
saturates), 35g carbs (33g
total sugars), 1g fibre

1. Set aside 12 cherries for the garnish. In a bowl, mix the remaining drained cherries with the cherry jam. Put the double cream, kirsch and icing sugar into a second bowl and use a hand-held electric whisk to lightly beat them together to soft peaks.

2. Crumble the brownies into 6 glasses or jars. Layer the cream and cherry mixture on top. Top each glass with a few brownie pieces and some of the reserved cherries. Sprinkle over the grated chocolate and serve.

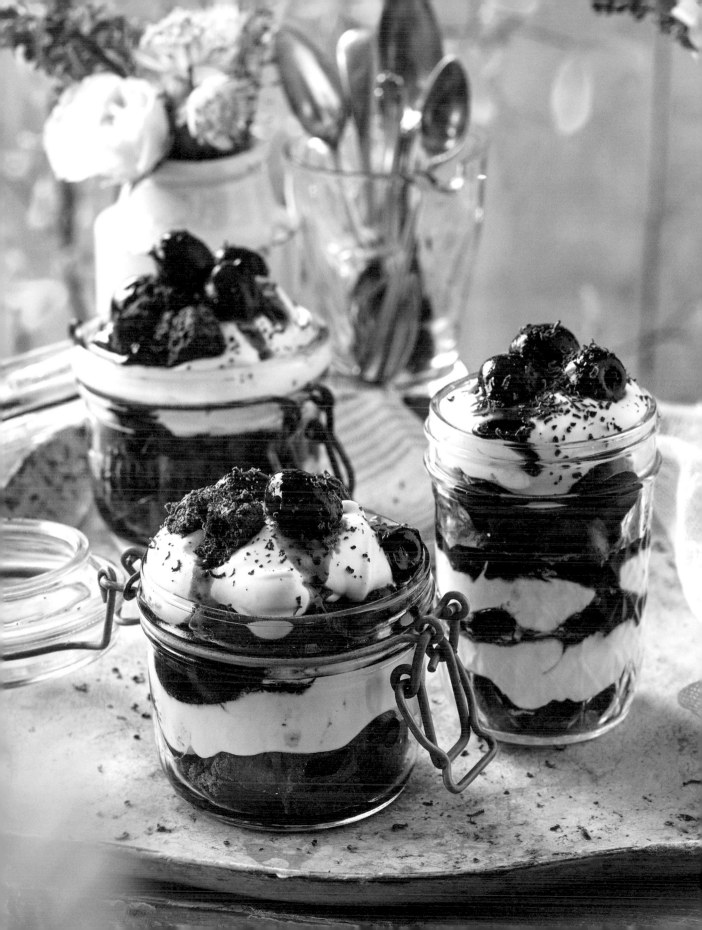

Chocolate Torte

This elegant cake would make a wonderful centrepiece for a special dinner or celebration.

Hands-on time: 15 minutes, plus 15 minutes chilling
Serves 8–10

200g (7oz) dark chocolate (70% cocoa solids), broken into pieces, plus extra, grated, to decorate
25g (1oz) butter, plus extra to grease
1 heaped tbsp golden syrup
200g (7oz) butter shortbread biscuits, finely crushed
40g (1½oz) icing sugar
300ml (½ pint) double cream
1–2 tbsp amaretto (optional)
Fresh raspberries, to decorate
Icing sugar, to dust
Crème fraîche, to serve

PER SERVING (for 10 servings) 409cals, 3g protein, 28g fat (17g saturates), 34g carbs (25g total sugars), 1g fibre

1. Melt the chocolate in short bursts in the microwave or in a heatproof bowl set over a pan of barely simmering water (don't allow the bowl to touch the water). Set aside to cool for 10 minutes.

2. Meanwhile, grease and line the sides of a 20.5cm (8in) loose-bottomed cake tin with baking paper. Put in the freezer to chill. Heat the butter and golden syrup in a pan until melted, then add the crushed biscuits. Mix well, then press the mixture into the base of the prepared tin. Return to the freezer to firm up.

3. Sift the icing sugar into a separate bowl. Pour in the cream and amaretto, if using, then whisk the cream using an electric hand whisk until it is thick but hasn't yet reached the soft peak stage. Briefly whisk in the cooled chocolate until combined and smooth – this won't take long, and the mixture will turn thick and mousse-like. Spoon the chocolate mixture into the cake tin, level the surface with the back of a dessertspoon, then cover and chill in the freezer for 15–20 minutes until set – for a firmer set, leave the torte for up to 1 hour.

4. Transfer the torte to a serving plate. Peel off the baking paper and scatter over grated chocolate. Dot over a few raspberries and lightly dust with icing sugar. Serve in slices with crème fraîche on the side.

◆ GET AHEAD
Make the torte to the end of step 3 up to a day ahead and chill overnight in the fridge instead of the freezer. Complete the recipe to serve.

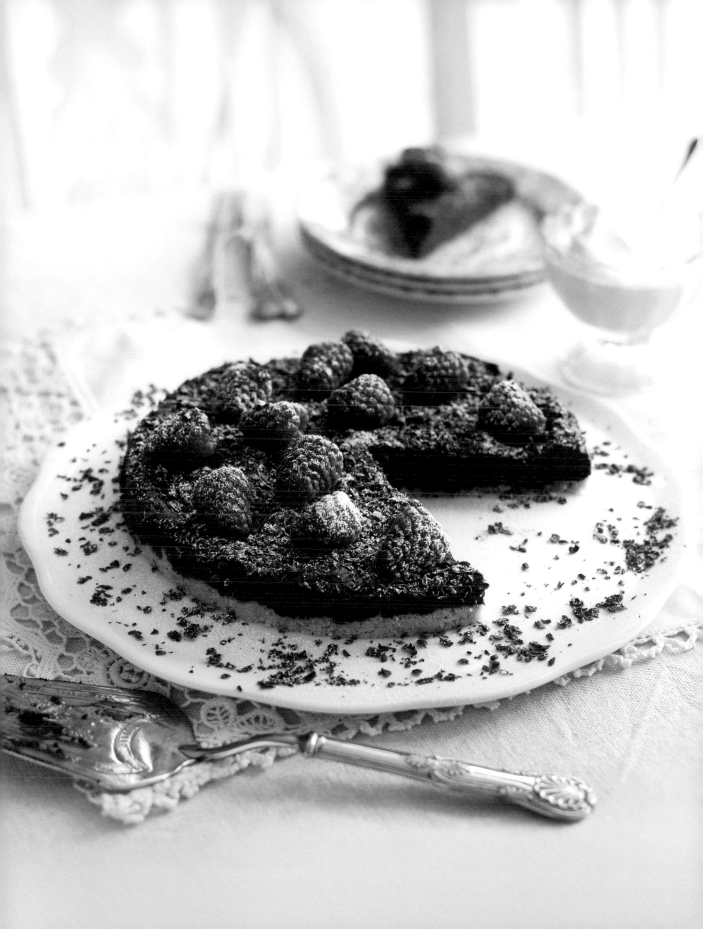

Blackberry Fool Cheesecake Tart

This truly is an instant showstopper and super easy to make. Mix up the berries, if you like, by using your favourites or mixed berries.

Hands-on time: 15 minutes
Serves 8

250g tub mascarpone
150ml tub double cream
100g (3½oz) natural yogurt
1 tsp vanilla bean paste or
    extract
Zest and juice of 1 lemon
3 tbsp icing sugar
100g (3½oz) blackberries
1 ready-made sweet
    shortcrust pastry case
    (about 20.5cm/8in)

PER SERVING 389cals,
4g protein, 31g fat (20g
saturates), 24g carbs (14g
total sugars), 1g fibre

1. Put the mascarpone, cream, yogurt, vanilla and lemon zest into a large bowl, then sift over 2 tablespoons icing sugar. Use a hand-held electric whisk to mix together until just stiff.

2. In a small food processor, whiz 50g (2oz) blackberries with the remaining icing sugar and lemon juice. Push the purée through a sieve (discard any pips), then marble through the creamy mixture.

3. Spoon the mixture into the pastry case, smooth into place and top with the remaining berries. Cut into slices to serve.

● GH TIP
For a gluten-free option, serve the cheesecake mixture in glasses or use a gluten-free pastry case.

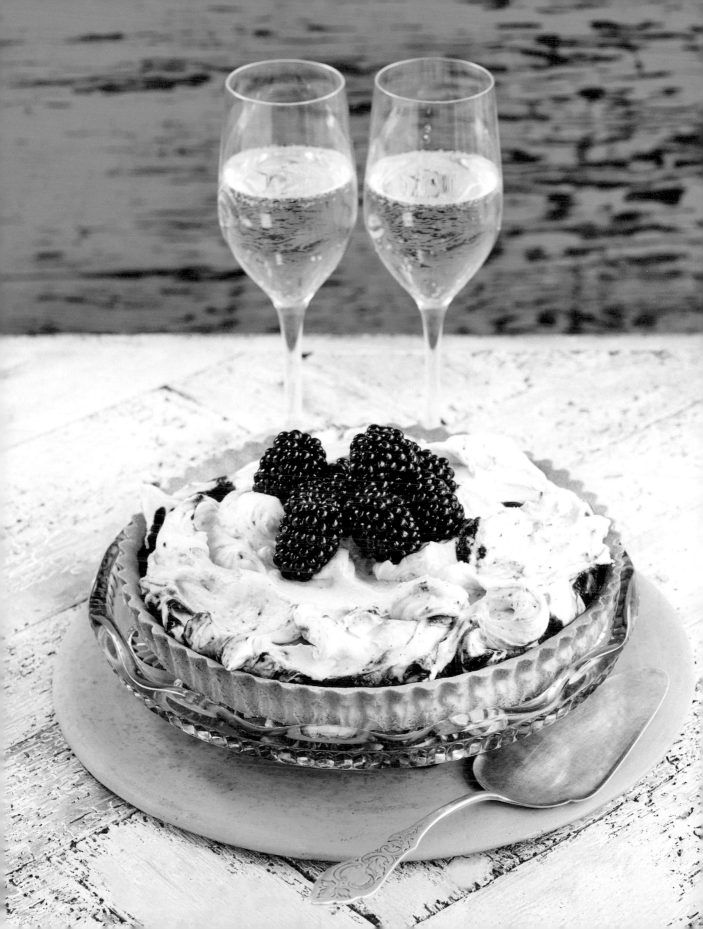

Jam Tarts

These super-simple strawberry tarts are a great choice when you're looking for something special to bring to a bake sale or office party.

Hands-on time: 10 minutes
Cooking time: 20 minutes
Serves 12

Plain flour, to dust
320g ready-to-roll shortcrust
   pastry sheet
175g (6 oz) strawberry jam

PER SERVING 118cals,
1g protein, 5g fat (2g
saturates), 16g carbs (10g
total sugars), 1g fibre

1. On a lightly floured work surface, unroll the pastry sheet. Use a 7.5cm (3in) fluted circle cutter to stamp out 12 rounds, then use a small heart-shaped cutter to stamp out 12 hearts.

2. Preheat the oven to 200°C (180°C fan) mark 6. Press the pastry circles into a patty tin, fill each with a rounded teaspoon of jam and bake for 10 minutes. Top with the hearts and return to the oven for 5–10 minutes until the pastry is cooked through.

3. Remove from the oven and allow to cool slightly before serving.

◆ GET AHEAD
Bake these ahead of time, ideally the day before you plan to serve them, then cool completely before transferring to an airtight container. They will keep for up to 4 days.

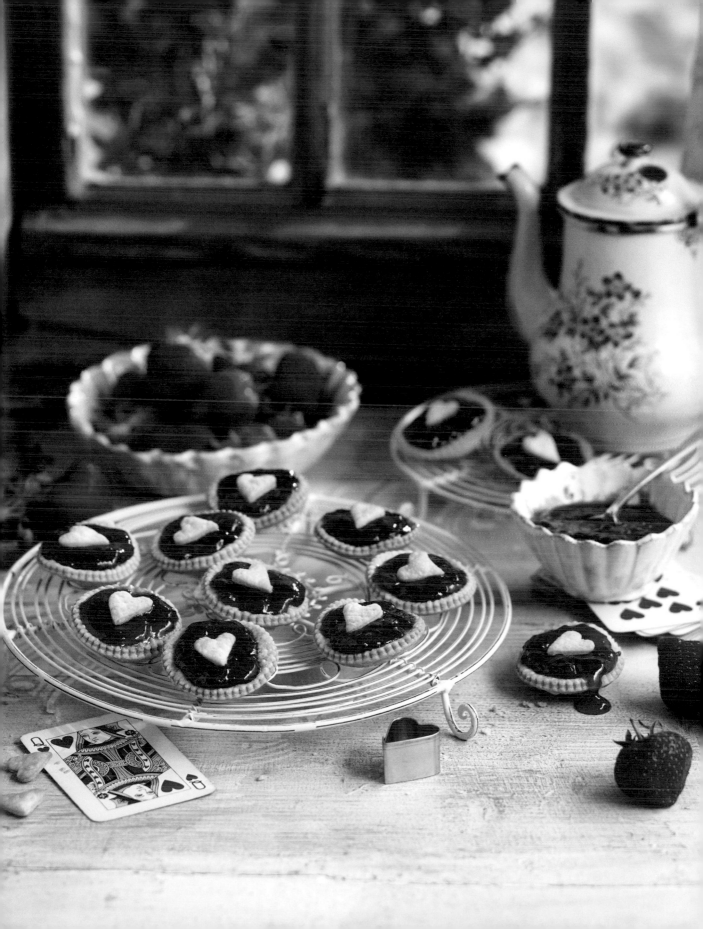

Peanut Butter Cookies

These quick cookies are the perfect treat. There are only three ingredients and they're free from gluten and dairy!

Hands-on time: 10 minutes, plus cooling
Cooking time: 12 minutes
Makes 18 cookies

250g (9oz) crunchy peanut butter
200g (7oz) light brown soft sugar
1 medium egg

PER COOKIE 135cals, 4g protein, 8g fat (1g saturates), 12g carbs (11g total sugars), 1g fibre

1. Preheat the oven to 180°C (160°C fan) mark 4. Line 2 baking sheets with baking parchment. Beat all the ingredients together in a medium bowl until well combined.

2. Scoop out tablespoons of the mixture and roll into balls. Arrange on the prepared sheets, spacing well apart. Press down with the back of a fork to flatten slightly.

3. Bake for 12 minutes, then leave to cool on baking sheet for 5 minutes. Transfer to a wire rack to cool completely. Serve.

Biscoff Traybake

A biscuit, turned into a spread, transformed into a cake. Sounds crazy, but this is probably the simplest bake you'll ever make. No scales, no whisk, no hassle!

Hands-on time: 5 minutes, plus cooling
Cooking time: 20 minutes
Makes 16 squares

400g jar Lotus Biscoff spread, plus 5 tbsp extra to decorate
3 medium eggs
2 tsp baking powder

PER SQUARE 158cals, 2g protein, 10g fat (2g saturates), 14g carbs (9g total sugars), 0g fibre

1. Preheat the oven to 180°C (160°C fan) mark 4. Line a 20.5cm (8in) square tin with baking parchment. Scoop all of the Biscoff out of the jar into a bowl, then add the eggs and baking powder. Mix together with a wooden spoon until combined.

2. Scrape the mixture into the lined tin and bake for 18–20 minutes, until just set. Leave to cool in the tin for 10 minutes, then evenly spread over the extra 5 tablespoons Biscoff spread. Cool, then cut into 16 squares.

● GH TIP
For extra texture, use smooth Biscoff Spread for the cake itself and the crunchy version for the topping.

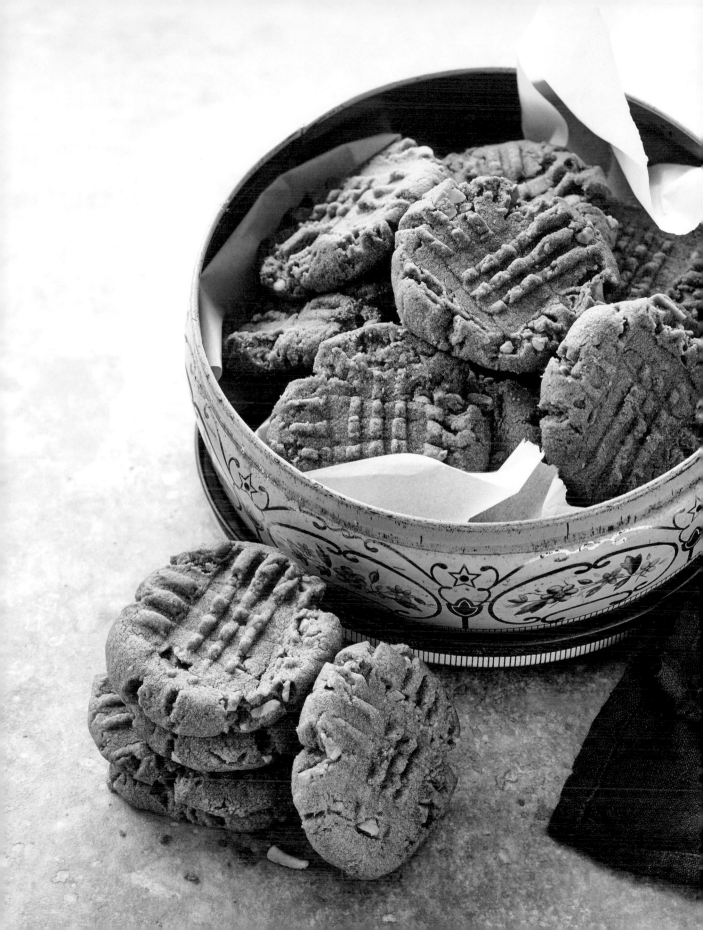

Chocolate Fondant Soufflés

There's always room for a classic chocolate fondant.

**Hands-on time: 15 minutes,
plus cooling
Cooking time: about
10 minutes
Serves 6**

100g (3½oz) unsalted butter,
chopped, plus extra
to grease
75g (3oz) caster sugar, plus
extra to dust
225g (8oz) dark chocolate,
chopped
2½ tbsp double cream, plus
extra to serve
5 large eggs at room
temperature, separated

**PER SERVING 475cals,
8g protein, 33g fat (19g
saturates), 35g carbs (35g
total sugars), 1g fibre**

1. Preheat the oven to 220°C (200°C fan) mark 7 with a baking tray inside (make sure there's space above the tray for the soufflés to rise). Grease 6 x 135ml (4½fl oz) ramekins with butter, then dust the insides with caster sugar, tapping out any excess. Chill the ramekins.

2. Gently heat the butter, chocolate and cream in a medium pan until melted. Remove from the heat and set aside to cool for 10 minutes. Gently stir in the egg yolks (don't overmix or the chocolate could seize).

3. In a medium bowl, whisk the egg whites to stiff peaks using a hand-held electric whisk. Add the sugar in one go and whisk back up to stiff peaks. With a large metal spoon, stir a spoonful of egg whites into the chocolate mixture to loosen it, then carefully fold in the remaining egg whites (being careful not to knock out the air).

4. Divide the mixture among the prepared ramekins. Level the tops with a palette knife, then run a knife around the inside of the rim (this helps to ensure a straight rise).

5. Carefully put the ramekins on to the preheated tray in the oven and bake for 9–11 minutes or until well risen. Serve immediately with extra cream, if you like.

◆ GET AHEAD
Make these soufflés up to a day ahead and chill them unbaked. Bake them for 12–14 minutes on a preheated tray to complete the recipe.

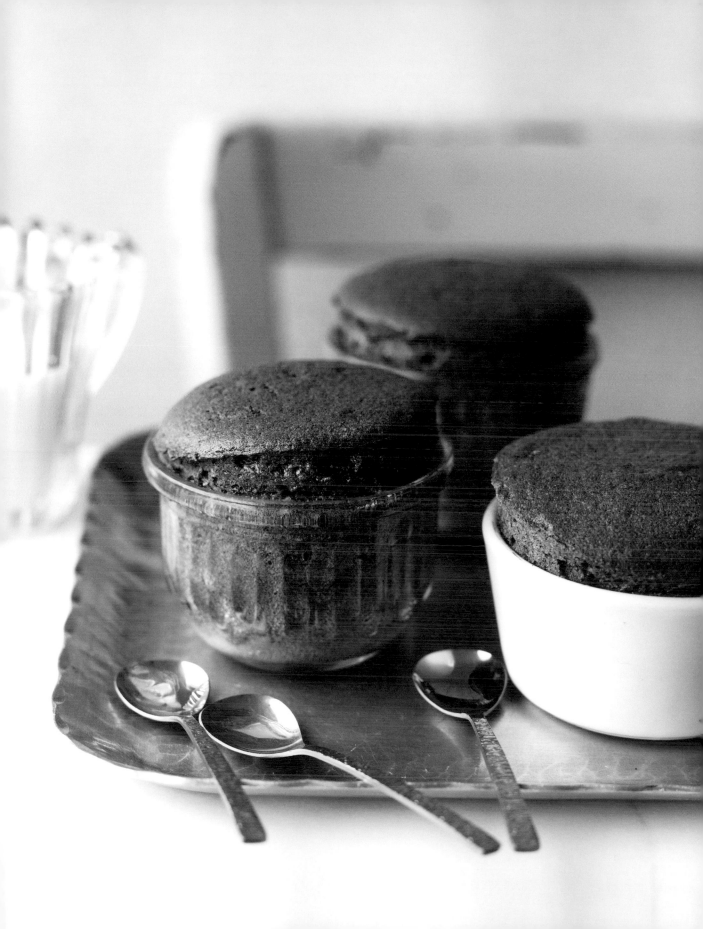

Strawberry and Limoncello Cheesecake Pots

These summery pots, with their lemony zing and strawberry sweetness, are quick to prepare and make an effortless yet impressive dinner-party dessert.

Hands-on time: 15 minutes, plus macerating
Makes 6 pots

200g (7oz) strawberries, hulled and quartered
75ml (3fl oz) limoncello
50g (2oz) icing sugar
250g tub mascarpone
150g (5oz) full-fat cream cheese
2 tsp vanilla bean paste
150g (5oz) amaretti biscuits
25g (1oz) toasted flaked almonds

PER SERVING 448cals, 6g protein, 29g fat (17.3g saturates), 36g carbs (35g total sugars), 1.3g fibre

1. Mix together the strawberries, limoncello and icing sugar in a bowl. Set aside and allow to macerate for 10 minutes.

2. With a hand-held electric whisk, gently beat together the mascarpone, cream cheese and vanilla bean paste until smooth. Strain the strawberries over a bowl and set aside. Add the strawberry liquid to the mascarpone mixture and beat to combine.

3. Put the amaretti biscuits in a food bag and use a rolling pin to lightly bash them into large crumbs. Divide the crumbs among 6 x 250ml (9fl oz) glasses, reserving about 2 tablespoons of the biscuit pieces to decorate. Spoon the mascarpone mixture over the biscuits, then top with the strawberries, a sprinkling of almonds and the reserved biscuit crumbs.

◆ GET AHEAD
Prepare the pots up to 4 hours in advance and keep in the fridge until ready to serve.

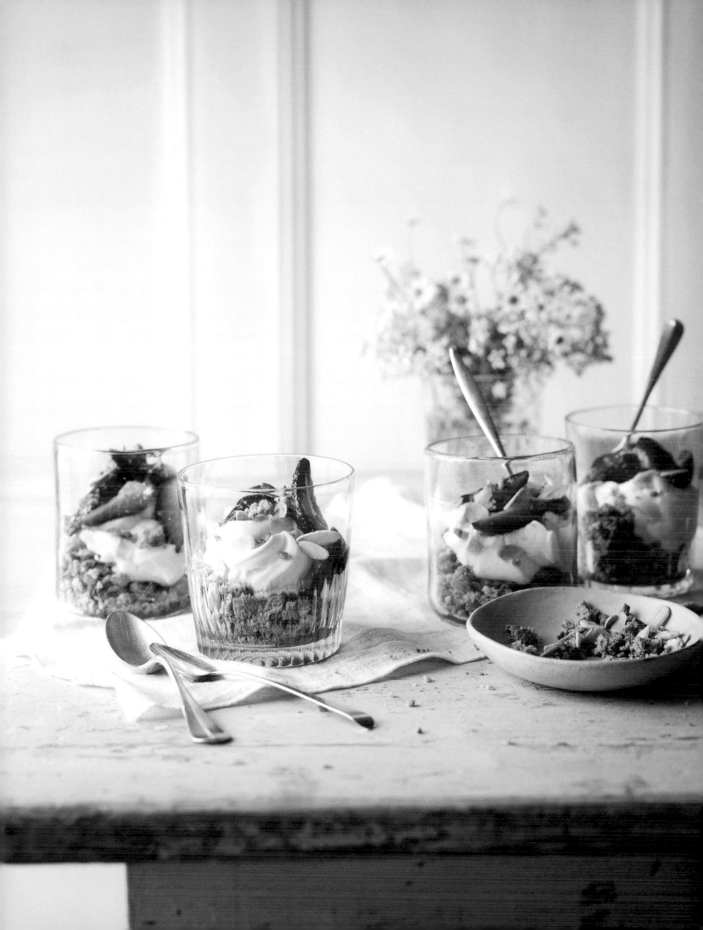

Copacabana Fruit Salad

This fruit salad is the ultimate party pleaser — serve the boozy syrup on the side so that guests can help themselves.

Hands-on time: 10 minutes, plus chilling
Cooking time: 5 minutes
Serves 8

2 tbsp sugar
Juice of 1 lime
1½ tbsp Malibu or white rum
1 pineapple, peeled and thinly
   sliced
1 large mango, peeled,
   destoned and sliced
1 melon, peeled, deseeded and
   chopped
2 passion fruit, halved

PER SERVING 72cals,
1g protein, 0g fat (0g
saturates), 14g carbs (14g
total sugars), 2g fibre

1. Put the sugar, lime juice and 1 tablespoon Malibu or white rum in a small pan set over medium heat. Stir until the sugar has melted, then bring up to the boil and bubble for 1 minute. Strain the syrup into a serving jug, stir through the remaining alcohol and chill.

2. Layer the prepared fruit on a serving platter and serve with the syrup alongside, allowing people to drizzle it over themselves.

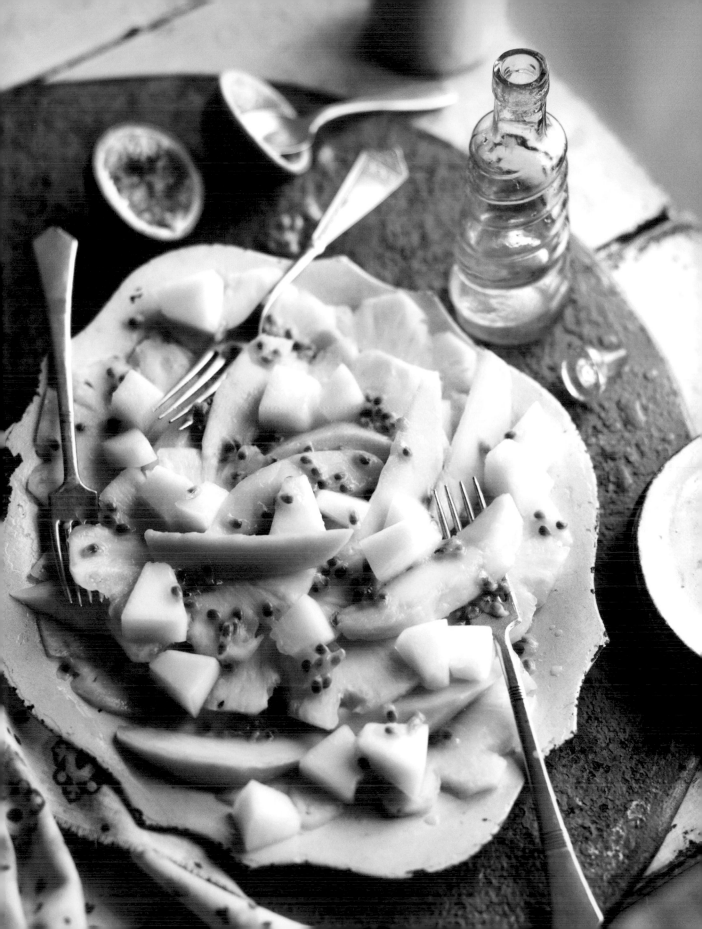

Mini Key Lime Pies

A creamy, rich filling flavoured with tangy citrus has made this pie a classic in the southern United States, and it's become a popular pud in Britain, too.

Hands-on time: 12 minutes
Cooking time: about
   5 minutes
Serves 4

2 sheets gelatine
150g (5oz) digestive biscuits
75g (3oz) butter
Zest and juice of 4 or 5 juicy
   limes – you'll need about
   125–150ml (4–5fl oz) juice
300ml (½ pint) double cream
397g tin condensed milk
12 lime jelly sweets, to
   decorate (optional)

PER SERVING (without sweets) 336cals, 4g protein, 24g fat (14g saturates), 26g carbs (20g total sugars), 1g fibre

1. Put the gelatine in a small bowl of cold water and leave to soak for 5 minutes. Meanwhile, whiz the biscuits in a food processor to form crumbs, (or put them in a freezer bag and bash them gently with a rolling pin until they resemble breadcrumbs). Melt the butter in a medium pan and stir in the crumbs. Line a 12-hole muffin tin with 12 muffin cases, then press a little of the crumb mixture (about a tablespoon) into the base of each case. Chill in the freezer for 5 minutes.

2. Heat half of the lime juice in a small pan until boiling. Remove the gelatine from the water, squeeze it out and add to the hot lime juice, stirring to dissolve. In a large bowl, whisk 250ml (9fl oz) of the cream with the remaining lime juice until thick but not yet at the soft peak stage. Add the condensed milk and gelatine mixture, then whisk until combined. Fold the lime zest into the mixture. Spoon the lime filling into the cupcake cases on top of the biscuit base. Chill in the freezer for 15–20 minutes or until set – for a firmer set, leave them in the freezer for up to 1 hour.

3. Whip the remaining cream to soft peaks, then drop a spoonful on top of each pie and decorate with lime jellies, if you like.

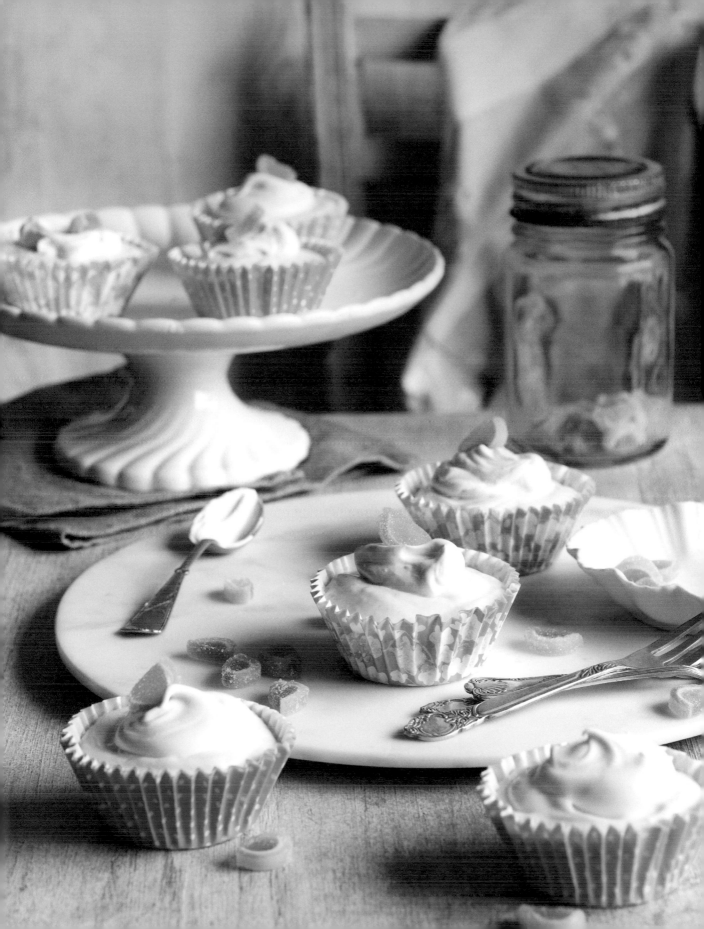

Tropical Eton Mess

Ready-made meringue kisses are a handy storecupboard standby — not to mention they're perfect for whipping up a quick Eton mess!

Hands-on time: 20 minutes
Serves 6–8

150ml (¼ pint) whipping
  cream
1 tbsp vanilla bean paste
500g tub 0% fat Greek yogurt
2 tbsp icing sugar
1 lime
300g (11oz) fresh mango
  pieces
4 passion fruit
1 papaya, peeled and sliced
25g (1oz) coconut flakes,
  toasted
About 30–40 meringue kisses,
  depending on their size

PER SERVING (if serving 8)
225cals, 8g protein, 9.75g fat
(6.75g saturates), 25g carbs
(25g total sugars), 2.25g
fibre

1. In a large bowl, whip the cream and vanilla paste until just stiff. Fold through the yogurt, sift over the icing sugar and mix well. Chill until ready to serve.

2. Zest the lime on to a plate lined with a damp kitchen towel, then cover it and put it in the fridge to prevent it from drying out.

3. Whiz half the mango and lime juice in a food processor until smooth, add the passion fruit pulp and pulse again to loosen the seeds. Pass the mixture through a fine sieve into a bowl and discard the seeds.

4. To serve, divide half the yogurt mixture among 6–8 glasses, add a few of the meringue kisses to each glass and drizzle with 1 tablespoon passion fruit sauce. Repeat with the remaining yogurt mixture, a few more meringue kisses, mango and papaya pieces, sauce, toasted coconut and the lime zest.

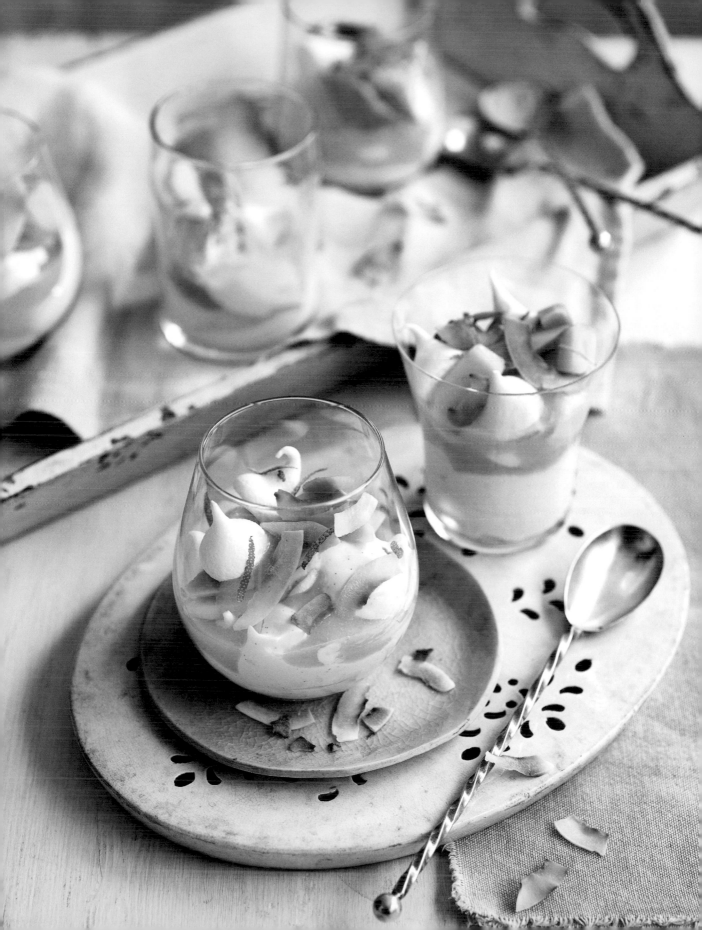

Rum, Banana and Ginger Ice Cream Sundae

Bananas, sticky rum sauce and ginger cake turn this sundae into a warming winter treat.

Hands-on time: 12 minutes
Cooking time: about
   5 minutes
Serves 4

50g (2oz) unsalted butter
150g (5oz) dark brown
   muscovado sugar
1½ tsp ground ginger
75ml (3fl oz) dark rum
Juice of 1 lime
125g (4oz) Jamaican ginger
   cake, cut into 8 slices
2 bananas, sliced
400ml (14fl oz) vanilla ice
   cream
4 physalis, to decorate
   (optional)

PER SERVING 620cals,
6g protein, 25g fat (13g
saturates), 81g carbs (71g
total sugars), 2g fibre

1. In a small saucepan, melt together the butter, sugar, ginger, rum and lime juice. Bubble for 5 minutes until it reaches a thick consistency and the sauce coats the back of the spoon.

2. Crumble 2 slices of ginger cake into each of 4 sundae glasses. Drizzle over 2 tablespoons rum sauce. Add a few banana slices, 2 scoops of ice cream and finish with more banana slices and another drizzling of rum sauce. Top with a physalis, if you like, and serve.

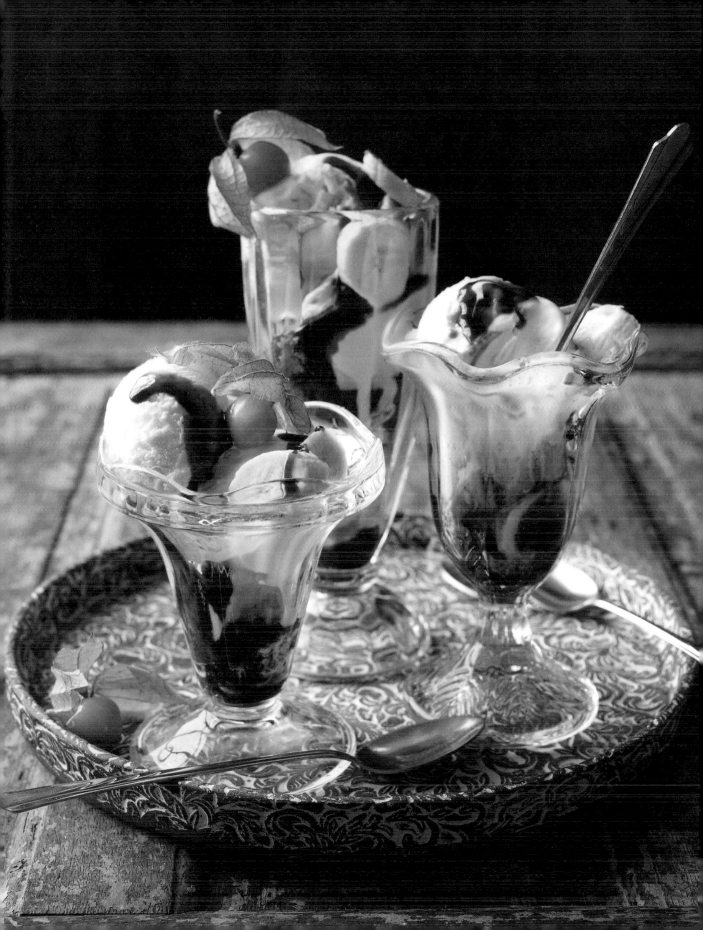

Index

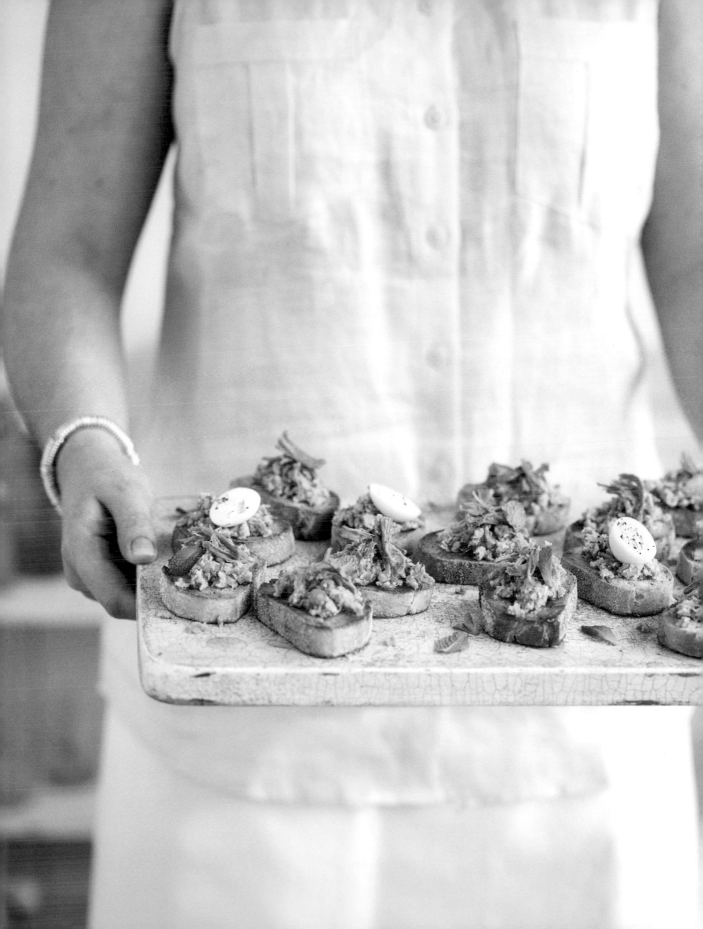